D1245310

Manual Therapy for Chronic Headache

Second edition

Joy Edeling BSc (Physio)
University of the Witwatersrand
Johannesburg
South Africa

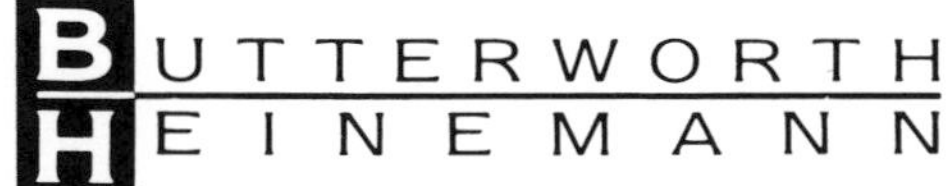

Butterworth-Heinemann Ltd
Linacre House, Jordan Hill, Oxford OX2 8DP

 A member of the Reed Elsevier group

OXFORD LONDON BOSTON
MUNICH NEW DELHI SINGAPORE SYDNEY
TOKYO TORONTO WELLINGTON

First published 1988
Reprinted 1990 (Twice)
Second edition 1994

© Butterworth-Heinemann Ltd, 1988, 1994

All rights reserved. No part of this publication may be reproduced in any material form (including photocopying or storing in any medium by electronic means and whether or not transiently or incidentally to some other use of this publication) without the written permission of the copyright holder except in accordance with the provisions of the Copyright, Designs and Patents Act 1988 or under the terms of a licence issued by the Copyright Licensing Agency Ltd, 90 Tottenham Court Road, London, England W1P 9HE. Applications for the copyright holder's written permission to reproduce any part of this publication should be addressed to the publishers

British Library Cataloguing in Publication Data
Edeling, Joy
Manual Therapy for Chronic Headache. –
2 Rev. ed
I. Title
616.0472

ISBN 0 7506 1619 9

Library of Congress Cataloguing in Publication Data
Edeling, Joy.
Manual therapy for chronic headache/Joy Edeling. – 2nd ed.
p. cm.
Includes bibliographical references and index.
1. Headache – treatment. 2. Physical therapy. I. Title.
RC392.E34 93–46472
616.8'4910622–dc20 CIP

Composition by Genesis Typesetting, Laser Quay, Rochester, Kent
Printed in Great Britain at the University Press, Cambridge

This book is dedicated to Geoff Maitland
from whose work it flows.

Contents

Foreword

Among the community in general, there are many people who have headaches which they accept as normal and they do not seek treatment; there is another group of people who also have headaches and who have sought treatment, but the treatment has been unsuccessful. The failures may have been because of wrong diagnosis or inappropriate treatment. This statement is not meant to be a destructive criticism, but rather a statement of fact. When people have nausea and vomiting as part of their symptoms they are often given a diagnosis of migraine or tension headaches. I doubt that anyone would disagree that tension can be a reason for headache, but not all tension headaches are due to tense muscles: rather the tense muscles have an effect on intervertebral segments and it is these which are responsible for the symptoms. When treatment makes the movements of the segment symptom-free, the end result is that, when the patient is under stress, he or she does not have a headache. In comparison with the number of people who have 'cervical' headaches the medical literature is so sparse as to be negligible. It is a pity that the books and articles that are written about headaches fail to give more than just a passing comment on the cervical spine as a source.

There are many reasons for this gap in our knowledge, one of which is that lay manipulations have been vigorous thus causing a worsening of the disorder and symptoms. The doctor is thus led to believe that 'manipulation' is a vigorous procedure, and that it can be harmful. I would hope that readers of this book would see that manipulation, as such, can mean extremely gentle techniques – and also that these gentle techniques can successfully clear or significantly improve a patient's headaches.

Although the mechanism of cervical headaches remains a subject of debate, the fact is that on examination, abnormally restricted cervical movements, when stretched or palpated as described in this book, can *reproduce* the patient's headache. This must surely indicate that headache must have some cervical spine component. Taking this one step further, if success is gained by mobilization treatment freeing both the movements and the headaches simultaneously this must mean that (1) cervical headaches are a diagnosable entity, and (2) treatment techniques to the cervical spine can relieve or free the patients of their headaches.

Finally, I would hope that the reader would see that careful and precise assessment both during a treatment session and from treatment session to treatment session is one of the essential aspects of successful treatment. The in-depth interpretation of the patient's story and the palpation findings on examination are also vital components.

G. D. Maitland, 1988

Author's note

Figures 8.5–8.11, 10.1–10.4 and 12.6 have been reproduced by kind permission from *Vertebral Manipulation*, 5th edn., G. D. Maitland, 1986, Butterworths, London; and Figures 8.12–8.14 from *Peripheral Manipulation*, 2nd edn., G. D. Maitland, 1977, Butterworths, London.

As my work on headache was built on Maitland's work on the spinal column his techniques of examination and of treatment are applicable in my text. These are so well described in his books *Vertebral Manipulation* and *Peripheral Manipulation* that I cannot improve on them and I reproduce them only for the convenience of the reader. It is important for the reader who is not familiar with the concept upon which this work is founded, to study the works of reference.

There are certain techniques and strategies which apply to the examination and treatment of headache more specifically than those of Maitland in which he considers the cervical spine in a more general way. And so, in this text there will be certain techniques taken verbatim from Maitland, others which I have modified and some which I have improvised. Technique should not be rigid and I have tried to show how important it is to find the therapeutic technique for a particular pain or other symptom comprising the cervical headache syndrome.

Please note: the convention of referring to the therapist as 'he' and the patient as 'she' has been used purely for convenience and no sexual stereotyping is implied.

Introduction to first edition

Cervical osteoarthrosis is a very common source of chronic headache, although in the past little attention was paid to it in the medical literature. It was usually the vascular migraine or the so-called tension headaches that were featured and only recently has there been a growing awareness of the significance of the cervical spine as a source of headache. The author, having long supported the latter view (Edeling, 1974), was encouraged recently to read a similar opinion expressed by Jull (1986a) who writes: 'It is suggested that the incidence of cervical involvement in benign headache could be underestimated. This may occur as there is considerable overlap in symptomatology between cervical headache, tension headache and, to a lesser extent, vascular headache.'

When the headache of cervical spondylosis is described, it is portrayed as being a rather vague and mild syndrome where the pain is confined to the occiput and is unaccompanied by migraine-like symptoms (Brain, 1963).

This description is correct, but the experienced clinician recognizes that this is merely the early stage of the syndrome. The fully developed condition, whether of degenerative or late post-traumatic osteoarthrosis, constitutes a very severe syndrome and is hard to distinguish from migraine as it shares many of migraine's associated symptoms such as visual disturbances, tinnitus, nausea and vomiting and is triggered by factors usually thought to trigger migraine only. It is a more disabling condition than migraine because there is seldom remission of pain and the severity of the pain is frequently comparable to that of migraine. These patients are dangerously dependent on drugs to enable them to get through each day.

Other writers such as Trevor-Jones (1964) and Maigne (1976) describe the cervical headache as being a more severe and complicated condition but they have not modified the image established by Brain (*Brain's Clinical Neurology* was, for many years, a standard textbook for medical students). The profile of the cervical articular headache described by Brain does not compare with the more advanced condition we see. The fully developed syndrome is thus seldom recognized by doctors for what it is.

Other factors which contribute to misdiagnosis could be that the neuro-anatomical basis is not generally understood and therefore the bizarre symptoms do not seem reasonable. Most commonly, because it is triggered by stress, it is diagnosed as a tension headache. It should be stressed here that tension headache and the headache which arises from cervical joints are one and the same thing. The reason that traditional treatment for tension headache so often fails is that all the medical textbooks and other literature prescribe treatment aimed at the muscle contraction, which is secondary to the joint lesion. The primary source of pain therefore goes untreated.

It then becomes a problem and the patient is referred for specialist investigation to exclude other causes. When no organic cause can be found and the patient does not respond to psychiatric treatment there seems to be nothing more that the medical establishment has to offer and the patient turns to lay practitioners and finally resorts to self-administered drug abuse.

Doctors have not traditionally thought of referring cases of chronic headache to physiotherapists and, when they do, it has been with a request to massage and apply heat therapy with a view to relaxing the muscle spasm which is thought to be causing the headaches. But in the cases where the pain derives from painful intervertebral joints and not primarily from the spasm of the muscles, such treatment will be only palliative and will not interrupt the course of the syndrome. However if the causative joint or joints are identified and mobilized with appropriate techniques, dramatic and immediate pain relief can be obtained. Although the headache will recur, possibly soon after the treatment, the positive response will indicate that this headache, which had not responded to potent analgesia, will respond progressively to mobilization therapy and it remains only to repeat the treatment, daily at first and then, as remission periods increase, less frequently until the patient is quite free of headache. The patient is then discharged and asked to report recurrences. This form of treatment greatly reduces or obviates the need for analgesics or any other form of medication, e.g. antidepressants and muscle relaxants.

Case history

A typical case of a cervical headache is that of a middle-aged man who had been suffering frequent prefrontal headaches for the past 10 or 12 years. The headaches had increased in periodicity and severity during the latter years and at presentation they had been present every day for the foregoing 18 months. He had stopped taking pain killers because even four compound analgesics taken together had no effect.

The headaches were triggered or aggravated by any activity which needed concentration, for example his daily work as a clerk, by watching television for any length of time, by long car trips (roughly 100 km), sharp light, noise and when he got angry. Associated symptoms were nausea, dizziness, a blurring of vision and tinnitus.

He had been examined over the years by many doctors and had been hospitalized on one occasion many years before for investigation and treatment specifically for headache. He could not remember what tests were done then but in later years he was examined by a neurologist who ordered a brain scan and an EEG. No abnormality was detected. His neck was then manipulated under anaesthetic but this did not alter the course of the headaches which continued to worsen.

He was referred for physiotherapy reassessment by an orthopaedic surgeon who diagnosed cervical spondylosis. X-rays were sent with the patient to demonstrate the condition.

On examination

Cervical physiological movement

Flexion and extension both appeared to be of full range and pain-free, but the application of pressure at the end of range produced sharp suboccipital pain.

Rotation to the left was painful at three-quarters of normal range and rotation to the right at half range. Left and right side flexion were also painful at three-quarter range.

Palpation for localized passive or accessory intervertebral movement (see Chapter 8)
Postero-anterior pressure over the occipito-atlantal joints on both sides was painful to slight pressure and also over the atlanto-axial joints, both centrally and paravertebrally. Before treatment was commenced it was established that the pain was present in the prefrontal area.

Treatment

Oscillating pressures over the occipito-atlantal joint (5 × Grade II postero-anterior passive intervertebral pressures according to Maitland) reduced the pain. The same pressures applied to the atlanto-axial joints relieved the headache altogether.

The headache returned about two hours later and when it returned it was less severe than it had been before. After the second treatment the headache was gone for 24 hours. After the third treatment the headache stayed away for a week and when he had been free of headache for two weeks he was discharged and asked to report subsequent recurrences, which he has not done to date, six months later.

Comment 1. Note that, although this headache was easily cleared up by means of the application of very gentle mobilizing techniques, it did not respond to manipulation under anaesthetic. The reason for this is most likely to be that a gross regional wrenching of the cervical spine failed to include the upper cervical joints which was the pain source. It is most unlikely, in a regional manipulation, that the atlanto-occipital joint will be moved in a therapeutic way.

Comment 2. Very few radiological studies of sufficiently good quality are found to demonstrate the presence or absence of osteoarthritic changes at the craniovertebral levels, which are the most common sites of the headache lesion. They are hardly ever reported on by the radiologist unless he is looking for an overt fracture or subluxation. It is most often assumed that cervical headaches arise at lower levels, and when surgery was performed to affect headaches, as was the fashion some years ago, it was invariably the C5/C6/C7 levels which were fused or decompressed. Thus, as is the case at other intervertebral levels, the presence or absence of demonstrable osteoarthritis is not a useful diagnostic feature. Far more relevant information is to be found in a well-taken subjective and objective clinical examination. Friedenberg and Miller (1963) wrote, in this connection: 'This similarity between symptomatic and asymptomatic groups throws considerable doubt on the value of roentgenograms as a basis for determining the degree of clinical severity of cervical degenerative disease.' Jull (1986b) observed: 'The upper cervical spine is a complex structure. . .'. The complexity of its movements has received extensive in vitro study but at present there is not a clinically applicable radiographic technique to demonstrate the complexity of normal or abnormal movement at the upper cervical joints. Neither is it possible to ascertain whether these joints are symptomatic or otherwise from radiographic techniques alone.'

Comment 3. Although there will be therapists who are able to relieve cervical headache by means of heat and massage, and others by means of the forceful manipulative thrust, the author is of the opinion that the therapeutic effect of treatment using gentle passive oscillating techniques is more enduring. This treatment leads to progressive improvement and de-escalation of the syndrome and the expected outcome, in even the severest cases, is the return to an occasional headache which most people regard as being a 'normal headache'. Few people are quite headache-free.

The majority of cervical headaches respond predictably, but there will be some which do not.

Clinical trials

This study was begun in 1971 when, after completing a course in vertebral manipulation given by Maitland the author found that many chronic headaches which had proved to be resistant to other forms of treatment, progressively abated when the newly learned method and technique was applied to the upper cervical spine. Two years later the results were analysed and published in the *South African Journal of Physiotherapy* (Edeling, 1974). They were as follows:

Cases treated: 105

Of these: 95 responded with prompt relief of pain and other symptoms
10 did not respond favourably or at all

These cases were followed up 6–12 months later.

Of these: 37 were able to be contacted
12 reported no recurrence of symptoms
17 reported significant sustained improvement
8 reported no sustained improvement

Overall: 78% responded
22% did not respond

There could be several reasons for poor response. One is that, although there might be cervical signs, the primary pathology lies elsewhere in which case it would be out of our field. There could be concurrent pathology which renders the manipulative therapy ineffective, e.g. an inflammatory component. It could also be of psychogenic origin, but it is unwise to jump to this conclusion just because we are unable to help it.

However, most often we could help the poor responders if we had more knowledge, skill and experience. We should not abandon them too soon. It will be evident from their history that we probably represent their last and only hope of being released from unrelenting pain (*see* Chapter 12).

In 1975 further results were analysed and published in the *Proceedings of the Jubilee Congress of the South African Society of Physiotherapy* (Edeling, 1975), which was later updated for inclusion in a multi-author book, *Modern Manual Therapy of the Vertebral Column* (Grieve, 1986).

Cases treated: 268

Of these: 163 were able to be contacted for follow up
120 reported no recurrence
14 maintained significant improvement
29 reported no sustained improvement

Overall: 82.2% responded to mobilization of the cervical spine
17.8% did not respond

At the time of going to press the number of cases seen and treated by the author is approaching 3000. Although subsequent results have not been published they maintain of the same order as those of the first two trials.

The fact that so many chronic headache cases, which had resisted all other forms of treatment, cleared up when the cervical spine was mobilized suggests that:

1. The pain source was to be found in the joints because a treatment which improved the joint condition caused the pain to abate.
2. The syndrome had not been recognizable for diagnostic purposes because it has not been adequately documented. Many writers describe a headache which is referred from the cervical spine but they usually show it as being a mild condition. It is the author's experience that this headache is only mild in the early stages. When the pathology progresses as a result of repeated or superimposed trauma or other unfavourable circumstances, it becomes a very severe condition. The fully developed syndrome is not identified in medical writing and because, clinically, it resembles the more familiar vascular migraine it is often diagnosed as such. Migraine drugs, however, are quite ineffective.

References

Brain, R. (1963) Some unsolved problems of cervical spondylosis. *British Medical Journal*, **1**, 771

Edeling, J. (1974) Migraine and other chronic headaches. Preliminary report on experimental physical treatment. *South African Journal of Physiotherapy*, **30**, 2–3

Edeling, J. (1975) The abandoned headache syndrome. *Proceedings of the Jubilee Congress of the South African Society of Physiotherapy*, 285–298

Friedenberg, Z. B. and Miller, W. T. (1963) Degenerative disc disease of the cervical spine. A comparative study of asymptomatic and symptomatic patients. *Journal of Bone and Joint Surgery*, **45**, 1171–1178

Grieve, G. P. (1986) *Modern Manual Therapy of the Vertebral Column*. Churchill Livingstone, Edinburgh

Jull, G. A. (1986a) Headaches associated with the cervical spine – a clinical review. In Grieve, G. P., ed., *Modern Manual Therapy of the Vertebral Column*, Chapter 30, Churchill Livingstone, Edinburgh

Jull, G. A. (1986b) Clinical observations of upper cervical mobility. In Grieve, G. P., ed., *Modern Manual Therapy of the Vertebral Column*, Chapter 29, Churchill Livingstone, Edinburgh

Maigne, R. (1976) An evocative and unexpected sign of cervical headache. Pain on pinch-rolling of the eyebrow. *Annales de Médecine Physique*, **XIX**, 7

Trevor-Jones, R. (1964) Osteo-arthritis of the paravertebral joints of the 2nd and 3rd cervical vertebrae as a cause of occipital headache. *South African Medical Journal*, **38**, 392–395

Introduction to second edition

Chronic headache

There are two disparate categories of the chronic headache condition:

1. Vascular migraine with its variants
2. Non-vascular daily headache.

These entities may present in the pure form or they may overlap to a greater or lesser extent.

Benign headaches, of which only 15–20% are thought to be vascular in origin, are reported to affect two-thirds of the population (Jull, 1981). The remaining 80–85% acquire various diagnoses, tension headache being the most frequently diagnosed and cervicogenic headache the least.

The pathophysiology of migraine is well documented and is a medically treatable condition. The pain mechanism involves vasodilation of cranial blood vessels and treatment is with vasoconstrictor drugs. In its pure form physical therapy has little to offer.

The second category is a subject of controversy. Because objective tests failed to show any pathology, and stress-related muscle contraction of the scalp and neck muscles seemed to be the only significant finding, this common non-vascular chronic headache came to be known as tension headache.

In 1962 the Ad Hoc Committee for Classification of Headaches published, in the *Journal of the American Medical Association*, a report to the effect that sustained muscle contraction of the head and neck muscles was the primary cause of this headache and therefore put forward the term 'muscle contraction headache' because 'tension headache', which had been used for years, seemed to imply that stress and nervous tension were the sole causes. Treatment directed at the tension, tranquillizers, as well as treatment for muscle contraction, muscle relaxants, heat and massage give disappointing results and introduce more drugs in a condition already at risk from drug overuse.

Although some EMG studies have demonstrated increased action potentials of the neck and scalp muscles which correlated with the headache, others have failed to show any specific correlation between the recorded muscle contraction and pain. Sustained contraction of these muscles has thus not been universally demonstrated in people suffering with this type of headache and so the term 'chronic daily headache' gained favour because it does not reflect the aetiology, which was poorly understood.

In 1988, a committee of the International Headache Society published an updated classification of headache disorders in *Cephalalgia*. It rejected the term 'muscle contraction headache' because the muscle contraction was not always present and called it instead, 'tension-type headache' until such time as more information on the pathogenesis is found.

In 1991, *Medical Clinics of North America* devoted a volume to 'headache', with Seymour Diamond MD as Guest Editor (Diamond, 1991). This volume serves as a convenient overview by world authorities on the subject and should represent the state of the art at that time. One contributor wrote about the tension-type headache, and I refer in particular to this thoughtful paper, 'Diagnosis and treatment of muscle contraction (tension-type) headache' by Robert S. Kunkel MD. The summary of this chapter reads as follows:

> 'Acute tension-type headache is a very common condition that rarely is a problem in treatment. Chronic tension-type headache, however, is often a difficult therapeutic problem. The pathogenesis is not well understood, but both peripheral muscle contraction and central pain modulating systems are probably involved. Therapy usually works best when multiple techniques are used, including pharmacologic, psychological and physiological modalities.'

The 1988 classification gives prominence to the tension-type headache but scant attention to the cervicogenic headache, and the volume cited above overlooks it altogether.

It is the contention of the author that there is no difference in the condition of tension-type headache and that of cervical headache. This hypothesis developed from the study of those chronic headaches which responded favourably to manipulative treatment of the upper cervical spine after failing to respond to any previous treatment. Those which responded positively to treatment by mobilization were considered to be the true cervical headache. The positive response to mobilization of cervical joints became the overriding diagnostic requirement. Nearly all of the proven cervical headaches had acquired a previous diagnosis of tension headache.

This book will show that the 'acute type' tension headache is the early cervical syndrome and the 'chronic' the fully developed cervical headache syndrome, and that the acute type becomes the chronic in time.

Manipulative therapists should not be diverted from cases bearing a diagnosis of tension headache but should evaluate and treat them as detailed in this book.

References

Ad Hoc Committee For Classification of Headaches (1962) *Journal of the American Medical Association*, **79**, 717–718

Diamond, S. ed. (1991) *Medical Clinics of North America. Headache*, **75** (3)

Headache Classification Committee of the International Headache Society (1988) Classification and diagnostic criteria for headache disorders, cranial neuralgias and facial pain. *Cephalalgia*, **8** (Suppl. 7)

Jull, G. (1981) Clinical manifestations of cervical headache. In *Proceedings of a Symposium on Cervical Spine and Headache*, pp. 28–42. Manipulative Therapist's Association of Australia, Brisbane

Kunkel, R. S. (1991) Diagnosis and treatment of muscle contraction (tension-type) headache. In Diamond, S. guest ed., *Medical Clinics of North America. Headache*, **75** (3), 595–603

1

What headache patients suffer

People who have an occasional headache have no conception of the martyrdom suffered by victims of the fully developed cervical headache syndrome. Cruel and persistent pain and its sequelae comprise an incapacitating condition for people who are otherwise healthy and strong.

Although pain is the dominant symptom it is not the only nor the most distressing one. It is common for these patients to experience bizarre and alarming accompanying symptoms such as visual disturbances, tinnitus, nausea and vomiting, epigastric pain, dizziness, disorientation, dysphasia, ataxia and more.

As a direct result of prolonged pain the following factors also become manifest:

Loss of concentration and intellectual function

School children fail examinations because of headache. Workers may lose their jobs, businessmen lose contracts, teachers prepare lessons poorly, housewives cannot cope with the running of their homes.

Depletion of mental and physical stamina

Pain in itself is a stressful and exhausting experience. When the enervating effect of loss of sleep and analgesic overuse is added to the pain, the headache sufferer becomes unable to function normally and becomes depressed.

Loss of vitality and diminished concern for others

Headache sufferers become immersed in their pain. They are unable to engender enthusiasm as they are accustomed to having their plans thwarted by headache. They are unwilling to commit themselves in any way in case the headache will oblige them to break the commitment. They live from day to day, making frantic use of the good days in order to make up for the lost days. They turn inwards upon themselves and lose sight of the interests of those around them. They become isolated and cast aside, losing touch with life due to lack of interest.

Lowered stress tolerance and irritability

This leads to a breakdown in interpersonal relationships. The spouse with a headache is short tempered and unpleasant to live with. Even if she stops complaining she remains a martyr and her husband becomes weary of the strain placed on ordinary family life. He is as frustrated as she by the fruitless quest for cure. Children are neglected by a headache-suffering parent and the other parent is obliged to take on additional responsibilities and chores. Children are obliged to lead an unnaturally quiet and docile life so as not to upset mother and so bring on or aggravate a headache. They may not bring their friends to play. They live a subdued life and are torn between impotent sympathy and resentment.

Relationships in all other spheres suffer too, whether at work or at school and social life is avoided or neglected. No-one wants that old frump at a party dampening it with her long-suffering air. I remember the wife of a popular public figure. Although she attended functions with her husband she was not liked because of her apparent aloofness. It was only when she came to me for help for her dreadful headaches that I realized that her manner was not one of arrogance but of a valiant attempt to bear up until she could go home to rest. Once her headaches were brought under control she began to enjoy her social obligations and soon became as popular as her husband.

Headaches in children

Children who suffer chronic headaches also inflict suffering on their parents. Parents will pursue every avenue in order to have the condition investigated and cured. When test after test reveals no organic cause, as is commonly the case, they become frustrated and if the headache continues to worsen and to restrict the child's normal activities, the parent feels desperate. At this stage one of the doctors they have consulted might have suggested that the child is using the headache to avoid school or some other unpleasant duty. Now the confused parents vacillate between sympathy, guilt and anger, often harshly disciplining the child in case she is having them on. The unfortunate child, who really is having bad headaches – as bad as any adult victim – and suffers no less from their sequelae, is in a helpless situation.

Case history

A 12-year-old girl had suffered a continuous moderate to severe headache over a period of four years. She had spent eight days in hospital undergoing tests which included a brain scan. No abnormalities were detected. A tentative diagnosis was put forward, that of classic migraine but no migraine-specific drugs had been prescribed. Four different analgesic compounds had been prescribed but as none had had any effect at all, medication was stopped.

Because the child's parents had been divorced at about the time of the onset of the headaches it was thought that she could be stressed and missing her father. She was referred to a psychiatrist who investigated this possibility but found her to be psychologically normal and well adjusted to the divorce. When no further help seemed to be forthcoming from the medical fraternity, her mother took her to a chiropractor on the advice of a friend. The first manipulation gave her relief that lasted seven days, but subsequent sessions did not have any beneficial effect. After 17 more sessions this treatment was abandoned.

The child was brought along as a patient on a short headache course which I was conducting some years ago. Subjective examination revealed that at about the time of the onset of the syndrome, four years previously, she had been hit on the head with a hockey stick. Prior to that incident she had never experienced a headache. She appeared to be an apathetic child without energy or drive. Her school work was poor and she was thought to be lazy. She did not like to read or run about and play. Further questioning, however, showed that she longed to play sport but each time she tried she had to drop out because it made her headache worse and so she stopped trying. When the headache was very bad it was accompanied by nausea and vomiting. She also felt dizzy, her vision blurred and she saw 'little things that jump'.

On testing the passive intervertebral movement of the upper cervical spine, Grade I central postero-anterior pressure on C2, C6 and C7 was found to be extremely sensitive. The left paravertebral joints were also tender to Grade I postero-anterior pressures at these levels and this finding corresponded with the leftsidedness of the headache.

These joints were mobilized according to the principles to be described in this book and the headache progressively abated. When next I had contact with the physiotherapist who had treated her after the course, I learned that this young girl now played hockey for her school and was taking part in a gymnastics display being put on for their city's centenary. She excelled at Greek dancing and was generally blossoming at school. She still had an occasional headache which responded to the same treatment.

Headaches in work and recreation

Many recreational and work activities require a particular fixation of the head on the neck. This position needs to be maintained for prolonged periods to enable the eyes to focus on the object of the activity. If this happens to be an uncomfortable joint posture for the particular cervical lesion which is responsible for the symptoms it will invariably bring on a headache or worsen an existing one. If the activity is purely recreational the person can give it up although it would mean sacrificing the pleasure and relaxation it could otherwise have afforded. But where the activity is occupational and breadwinning there is no such escape possible and that person is obliged to make excessive use of drugs in order to get through the working day. There are few modern-day occupations which do not require a fixed head-on-neck posture for eye focus and concentration. Dentists, artisans, typists, bookkeepers and accountants, surgeons, artists, writers and businessmen who suffer headaches of cervical origin daily aggravate and perpetuate their pain in this way. This makes for strained relationships with their colleagues, bosses, employees and the public with whom they must deal. The telephonist who is rude and abrupt may be trying to cope with a splitting headache.

Outdoor recreation could become impossible for those whose headaches are provoked by bright sunlight and nightlife is restricted because they cannot tolerate noise or smoky rooms. Intolerance of rich foods and alcohol further curtail social life and holidays are best avoided because car travel worsens the pain.

The fruitless search for relief during which a great deal of time and money are spent leaves them with dashed hopes and also with the destructive effects of analgesic overdose. They face rejection by friends and family who grow weary of endless complaint or, alternatively, silent martyrdom. They come to understand from their doctors that either there is nothing wrong with them, or that they are producing their headache by means of excessive nervous tension. They understand that nothing more can be done and they do not know how to carry on. This leads to depression and self-doubt and a realization that they are regarded as hypochondriacs. They suffer deep anxiety over the possibility of undiscovered or undisclosed morbid pathology and this gives rise to even more stress.

The following is a follow-up report of a headache patient, a woman 50 years of age, whom I treated in 1977. Five years after this treatment she wrote:

> Until the age of 28 I was a gregarious person who loved entertaining and going out. Then I began to realize that having visitors or going to a show usually left me with a headache. I often woke with a headache. Sometimes it would wear off during the day but it could last for many days. I had accepted headaches as being part of my life since childhood. At first they were thought to be as a result of sinusitis and later of menstruation. When, at around the age of 30 they became more severe and more frequent I was told that they were caused by tension. I always seemed to be tired and looking back I see myself as a zombie, doing only what had to be done and going only where I was obliged to go. Everything was an effort and nothing was enjoyable. I tended to put off doing things until it was a good day and then would rush about trying to cram as much as I could into that day in case the next was a bad day. I was reluctant to make arrangements in advance and preferred to do things as the headache allowed. Most of the time I felt as if my brain and my eyes were covered by a veil and if only I could remove it everything would become clear to me. In a discussion I always felt as if I lost the thread. I couldn't concentrate however hard I tried. I often felt disappointed because when I wanted answers to questions I wasn't always able to formulate the questions.
>
> Pain set up a vicious circle. As I felt it coming on I would retreat inside myself. Nothing outside myself was real. I was unable to think of doing anything to help myself. It was only when the pain became less sharp that I would be able to do anything at all. My family didn't really regard me as a headache person, possibly because I seldom drew attention to my headaches. They saw me as a person with very low energy and who was antisocial.
>
> I can handle pain elsewhere in my body as long as my head is clear. But if my head aches I feel panicky in case the headaches should start up again. I feel as if I have missed out on life and want to make up for all those pain-filled years. I am enjoying life for the first time now since I was a child.

This woman is now studying for a degree and when she wrote this was in her third year of study. She sometimes comes for treatment for a thoracic ache at examination time but she no longer suffers from headache.

The object of this chapter is to bring home to the therapist the fallacy of the 'bored housewife syndrome'. Any practitioner who is unable to ease his patient's suffering is tempted to ease his own disappointment by supposing that the complaint is produced for a purpose and that the patient is reluctant to be relieved of it because it is serving some psychological end. I find this not to be true. These people are truly victims of a disabling condition. They are encapsulated in pain and prevented from following the lifestyle they would choose. This is evidenced by the enthusiasm with which they launch back into life once they have been released from perpetual pain.

I think that when medical practitioners are unable to relieve pain it does not mean that the pain is supratentorial but that we have not been able to pinpoint the source or have not found the right treatment. This fact is highlighted by the fact that the thousands of severe chronic headache syndromes who had been thoroughly investigated by medical specialists and not been helped, responded to a very simple procedure applied to the cervical spine.

2

Diagnosis of headache

Physiotherapists have not traditionally played a role, other than a palliative one, in the treatment of headache and even less of a role in the diagnosis. But in the development and advancement of manipulative therapy we have acquired a therapeutic potential to restore pain-free function to joints which is not only effective for backache but also for headache. The ready response of the tension-type headache to treatment by mobilization of the cervical spine leaves no room for doubt that it is in the cervical vertebral joints that the primary pain source is to be found. It is a diseased state of the cervicocranial joints that emits the head pain and not the muscle tension. Tension plays an important role but as a trigger, not the cause. These findings enable us to make a contribution to the diagnostic debate on chronic headache.

Headache accompanies many medical and surgical conditions but the primary pain mechanisms which can give rise to headache may be summed up as:

1. Vasodilation of cranial blood vessels as in migraine.
2. Non-migrainous vasodilation of cranial blood vessels induced by fever, drugs, hypoglycaemia, caffeine withdrawal, excess alcohol and other toxic conditions.
3. Traction on pain-sensitive intracranial blood vessels caused, e.g. by space-occupying lesions in the brain.
4. Local pain in a cranial structure, e.g. temporal arteritis or ocular, aural and dental pain, neuralgia and neuritides.
5. Pressure on or irritation of pain-sensitive structures which refer pain to the head, for example a painful condition of the upper cervical articulations or the temperomandibular joint. Muscle, neural and vascular tissue may be involved to a greater or lesser extent.
6. Pericranial muscle tension (no longer considered a prime cause). (Pikof, 1984; Chapman, 1986; Kunkel, 1991)

Mechanisms 1 and 5 are the most common ones responsible for the 'chronic (recurring) headache' syndromes.

Clinical observation and experience suggests to the author that an unnecessary distinction is made between mechanisms 5 and 6. Mechanism 5 produces the true cervicogenic headache and mechanism 6 produces the same headache in which muscle tension plays a prominent role but does not constitute a separate pathological entity. The craniocervical and upper cervical apophyseal joints constitute the primary pain source and tension, spasm or hyperactivity of the pericranial musculature contributes to the pain syndrome.

In the most recent classification of headache (Headache Classification Committee of the International Headache Society (HCCIHS) 1988), like those before it, a major section is devoted to the tension-type headache (HCCIHS, 1988i) with subheadings denoting episodic tension-type headache and chronic tension-type headache, each of which may be associated or unassociated with disorder of the pericranial muscles, as 'muscle contraction has not universally been demonstrated in persons suffering this type of headache' (Kunkel, 1991).

The only reference to a headache which could be of cervical joint origin is to be found in the Classification (HCCIHS, 1988), under the heading:

'*Headache or facial pain associated with disorder of the cranium, neck, eyes, ears, nose, sinuses, teeth, mouth or other facial or cranial structures*'.

Then, under a subheading entitled:

'*Neck*',

there is another subheading:

'*Cervical spine – Diagnostic criteria*'

and the diagnostic criteria supplied are inadequate and misleading.

Headaches that fall within the first four categories given above will not be seen by physical therapists as they do not fall within our field of endeavour. But the fifth and sixth group together form the true cervical headache and will respond to the treatment outlined in this textbook.

If we accept that 'tension-type' headache is really the true cervical headache, it is also necessary to know that the one termed 'episodic tension-type headache' in the 1988 Classification is in truth the early cervical headache syndrome and that the 'chronic tension-type headache' is the late or fully developed syndrome, and that the first becomes the second in time (*see* below).

If we wish to realize our potential in this field we must direct our efforts at the large percentage of the population that suffers from the so-called *tension headache*, because it is these that we will be able to relieve by means of mobilizing cervical joints.

Because these headaches respond so poorly to medical treatment and so well to gentle mobilization, manual therapists would do well to give them more serious attention. They constitute a huge field of work for us. We must learn how to recognize, assess and successfully treat them. We should also make doctors more aware of the fact that there is an alternative to the ever-increasing drug regimen. Cervicogenic headache is a biomechanical and not a medical problem and appropriate treatment is biomechanical rather than medical.

Differential diagnosis of chronic headache

The first differentiation necessary is to establish whether the headache is chronic (recurring), or whether it has evolved recently as a symptom of another systemic condition: if so, the patient should see a medical doctor for treatment of the condition.

If it is established that the headache is chronic the next step is to decide whether it is cervicogenic or vascular in origin. The first question should be: 'How often do you have headache?'. If the answer is 'once every three months' the probability is that it is migraine and if the answer is 'several times a week' it is more likely to be cervicogenic. This is followed, of course, by the line of questioning detailed in Chapter 7.

Diagnostic process

There seems to be no objective test or collection of symptoms which reliably points to the diagnosis of chronic headache. Rather it is the pattern, not only of the presenting symptom syndrome but of the way it has behaved over time since its onset. The natural history of the condition must be revealed through careful questioning. This is the most useful diagnostic exercise, and at the end of about 30 minutes of questioning it is possible to know whether the headache will respond to mobilization of the neck or whether it is migraine or the combined syndrome (*see* below).

Questioning is followed by physical examination from which the most useful information is gained by palpation of accessory movement of the craniovertebral joints (Chapter 8). Having identified the source in this way, very gentle mobilization of these joints reliably causes an existing headache to ease or to abate. This provides clinical confirmation of a tentative diagnosis of cervicogenic headache and one may confidently expect that repetition of the same technique on subsequent days will result in progressive abatement of the headache until its frequency and severity have been so reduced as to be acceptable. At this point a retrospective diagnosis is indisputable. Trial mobilization will prove to be the most reliable diagnostic procedure (*see* Case no. 8, Chapter 16).

Diagnostic profile of clinical presentation of cervical headache

The patient presents with frequent headache – at least three times per week and often daily or continuous. The intensity of the pain fluctuates from 1 to 5 on a 5-point scale. Upon questioning it is revealed that both the periodicity and the intensity of the pain have worsened over a long period, usually over many years. The response to analgesia has also worsened as the pain intensity increased.

The pain may be felt in any part of the head, unilateral, bilateral or alternating and often but not necessarily in the neck. The pain characteristic, when the pain is severe, is often described as throbbing or pounding and a feeling of pressure, either explosive (bursting) or compressive (crushing), is common. Piercing pain, a tight band round the head and a feeling as if the eyes are being pushed out are familiar descriptions. When the pain is severe it is accompanied by other symptoms such as nausea, vomiting, dizziness and visual and aural disturbances.

In most cases there is a history of head or neck trauma, often so long before the onset of the headache as to have been temporarily forgotten.

The headaches are triggered or aggravated by many factors, the most common being emotional stress and sustained occupational positioning of the neck. The stress need not be emotional tension but any circumstance which is irritating to that particular individual, e.g. cold, heat, glare or flashing lights, loud or discordant noise and many more such everyday encounters. It is unusual for the headache to be triggered or aggravated simply by a movement, as a backache may be by bending.

The patient will, by this stage, have consulted many medical specialists and it is typical that all diagnostic tests will have been negative and treatments failed. Previous therapy may also have failed where the therapist had directed treatment at the muscle tension or even at the cervical spine in a less specific manner than taught in this book, e.g. traction or regional manipulation or inaccurately applied mobilization.

If the pain is confined to the head and is not felt in the neck, physiological or active movement testing will reveal little or no restriction. It is only on palpation of accessory movement of the craniovertebral joints that the culpable joint will be identified. The very lightest pressure exerted there will be exquisitely sensitive and painful, often referring directly to the usual pain area in the head, so that the patient at once identifies it as the source of the headache and a few gentle pressures applied to this joint could instantly relieve an existing headache. This is not magic as the patient is inclined to suspect but treatment directed at the primary cause of the headache. Repeated treatments will result in progressive de-escalation of the chronic headache syndrome. The patient will spontaneously reduce and finally cease her drugs and concomitant depression will lift as the patient resumes her normal lifestyle.

The aim of the treatment should not be held up as a cure. The arthrosis is not reversible but is rendered subsymptomatic as it was before the symptoms escalated to the chronic state. Headaches which occur less than once a month are not severe and which abate from a simple analgesic are regarded by the general population as being normal. Recurrences should respond to the same treatment.

This is in essence the clinical presentation of the late stage of the uncomplicated cervical headache syndrome taken from over three thousand cases examined as described in this book and *which responded to mobilization.*

Headache and depression

It is generally accepted that depression can be the root cause of chronic pain where no organic cause can be found. But it is less well recognized that chronic pain can cause depression, especially if numerous attempts at diagnosis and treatment have been ineffective (*see* Chapter 1). We will see many cases where this has been the case and who are in a considerable state of depression when they are referred to us as a last resort. A significant number of these will prove to be undiagnosed headaches of cervical spondylosis which clear up readily when the upper cervical spine is mobilized. It is then very interesting to see the depression lift as the pain recedes, and the patient resumes her natural *joie de vivre* (*see* case history and follow-up report in Chapter 1).

Much is also written about the 'migraine personality' which is said to underly chronic headache, not only migraine but also tension headache (Frazier, 1964). The reader should study the description of this personality and then look about and try to identify it among acquaintances. Does everyone who is meticulous, perfectionist or compulsive suffer chronic headache? They do not, but if they have an upper cervical lesion, the stress-induced contraction of the cervical muscles will result in perpetual headache. But these can be relieved by treating the cervical lesion without needing to modify the personality. Also, if they are migraine-prone, these tense people will suffer more from migraine than a more phlegmatic migraine-prone person.

Headache of delusional, conversion or hypochondriacal states

Many of the cases which have responded readily to manipulation of the neck had previously been diagnosed as psychogenic headaches because the source of the headache in the cervical spine had been missed.

Physiotherapists think in terms of physical and mechanical concepts. We deal primarily with the hardware of the human body and psychiatrists could be said to deal in the software. But in most conditions the hardware and the software are not separable. In chronic headaches both these aspects are involved, each one influencing the other to a greater or lesser extent.

If chronic headaches were to be evaluated by a manipulative therapist before being referred to a psychiatrist, the dominantly mechanical headache of cervical spondylosis would be identified and treated. This would be more sensible because results from manipulation are more immediately obtained than from psychotherapy. Depending on the degree of the psychogenic component, we will obtain only partial success or no success at all. In such cases we would be grateful for a chance to consult with a psychiatrist and to refer the patient. Similarly, when patients who are referred for psychiatric evaluation are found to be psychologically normal (*see* case history in Chapter 1), or psychiatric treatment fails, it would be appropriate to call in the services of a manipulative therapist who has an interest in treating headaches.

It now remains to differentiate the vascular headache from the cervical articular headache (also known as tension headache).

Differential diagnosis of vascular migraine and fully developed cervical articular headache

Area of pain distribution

The area of pain distribution is not a reliable criterion for differentiation. Many headache sufferers diagnose their own 'migraine' simply because they have localized pain on one side of the head, whereas cervical headaches supposedly arise suboccipitally and spread over the occiput.

Headaches of cervical origin are not always occipital as is stated by Lord Brain (Brain, 1963), neither are they unilateral as claimed by Sjaastad (1983). In fact, occipital pain is often absent in cervical headaches and the pain can be referred to any part of the head whether unilateral, bilateral or alternating (Edeling, 1974; Jull, 1981). It occurs in many patterns, from a diffuse pain involving the whole cranium to localized areas as small as a needlepoint. Frequently a narrow line is described as arising suboccipitally, ascending over one hemisphere and settling in or behind one eye. But, equally commonly, the pain is felt to arise near the eye and to radiate posteriorly from there. A tight band compressing the skull is also commonly described by the sufferer of a cervical headache, as is central vertex pain, bi-or unilateral temporal, parietal, frontal, peri-orbital or perinasal pain. All of these are common referral areas from the upper cervical spine, although many authorities hold them to be typical of migraine. When the pain encroaches onto the face, however, it is often referred from the temporomandibular joint.

Furthermore, because a migraine sometimes involves the whole head, pain distribution alone is not a diagnostic feature.

Nature of pain

The pain characteristic is not a reliable feature for differentiating between cervical headache and migraine. A boring pain or one that throbs is too hastily labelled migraine, usually by the patient and sometimes by the doctor. According to Brain (1963), the cervical headache is not that sort of pain. The truth is that cervical headache presents with many pain characteristics, e.g. boring, throbbing, burning, a feeling of pressure, pounding, thundering, gnawing or sickening. Descriptions such as 'it feels as if my eyes are being pushed out' or 'as if a steel rod is being pushed through my brain' are not uncommon in cervical headache.

Total pain pattern

I have numerically assessed three features, Periodicity (P), Intensity (I) and Response to analgesics (R) in order to establish the severity of the total headache syndrome at presentation and to record its decline or otherwise during treatment and later when following it up (Edeling, 1980), *see* Chapter 7. Briefly, each of these factors is graded from 1/5 to 5/5 so that a total pain pattern score of, say 3/15, would denote a mild syndrome and one of 15/15 a totally insupportable condition. The behaviour of these three factors throughout the natural history of a chronic headache syndrome offers, perhaps, the most reliable way of subjectively distinguishing the cervical from the vascular headache.

Periodicity

A fully developed cervical headache displays a history of increasing periodicity. The patient remembers a time when she had 'normal headaches'. This usually means a headache of low intensity (I = 1/5–3/5), infrequent (P = 1/5) and totally relieved by a simple analgesic (R = 1/5) (TPP = 3/15–5/15). These headaches are called 'normal' by the patient because she thinks that everyone has such a headache under certain circumstances. Perhaps many people do have an early cervical headache which does not necessarily develop. Usually, by the time a headache patient seeks treatment the periodicity is high. A continuous headache (P = 5/5) with its intensity fluctuating from 1 to 5 is the typical syndrome of the fully developed cervical articular headache.

On the other hand, pure migraine is of low periodicity (P = 1/5–2/5) and it does not increase over the years. It is nearly always of maximum intensity (I = 5/5), with no intervening lower intensity headaches. Its pattern is established at the onset of the syndrome and hardly varies until it abates spontaneously in later life. The cervical headache does not abate in later life.

The bizarre periodicity patterns of the migrainous cluster headache and neuralgias are atypical in cervical headaches but do occur. Therefore this feature does not entirely rule out a cervical cause. Headaches of temporomandibular origin are also often of irregular periodicity. When a migraine headache becomes more frequent one may confidently suspect the intervention of a cervical component.

The pattern then is one of infrequent, very severe attacks of headache and also less severe headaches in between, which gradually become more frequent and severe.

Intensity of pain
It is a commonly held fallacy that the cervical headache is not as painful as migraine. This is not true. The only difference is that whereas a migraine always rates an intensity of 4/5 or 5/5, the cervical headache varies from 1/5 to 5/5 depending on the stage of the pathology and the potency of the precipitant.

Response to analgesics
I think that this factor is related to the intensity of pain experienced. In cervical headache simple analgesics become ineffective at a certain stage because the pain has become more severe. During the course of successful treatment of a cervical headache, analgesics which had previously had no effect once more become effective. Correspondingly, at this stage of the treatment the patient will have reported an overall decline in the periodicity. Hence decreasing response to analgesics also suggests a cervical origin. However, throughout its course migraine responds minimally to compound analgesics and not at all to simple analgesics.

Precipitating factors

Authorities agree that migraine is triggered by light, noise, smells, inclement weather, exercise, excitement, emotion and certain ingestants such as chocolate, cheese, coffee and wine and that cervical headaches are triggered merely by postural malpositioning.

From my sample (*see* Introduction to first edition) it is clear that cervical headaches can be triggered by nearly all the so-called migraine trigger factors. In addition to cervical malpositioning cervical headaches are set off by many other factors. If there is a dominant common factor it seems to be any stressful situation whether biological or emotional. If there is a difference, it seems to be that the migraine attack is sometimes unprecipitated, it just periodically 'comes out of the blue'. However, the fully developed cervical headache subject usually knows what precipitates or aggravates her headache. Of the precipitants, the ingestants are more commonly a factor in migraine, but alcohol often triggers a cervical headache. Both types can exacerbate premenstrually.

Associated or accompanying symptoms

In the literature so much is made of the accompaniments of migraine that when a severe headache presents with any of these it acquires a migraine label. On the other hand, although some writers have described similar symptoms related to cervical disorders (Trevor-Jones, 1964; Edeling, 1974; Jull, 1981), this does not seem to be widely known. The truth is that cervical headaches commonly display nearly all the associated symptoms thought to be diagnostic of migraine. In particular, visual disturbances, tinnitus, nausea and vomiting and dizziness are common.

However, there are differences in the way in which some of these common symptoms present. For example, although the cervical headache is often accompanied by visual disturbances at the height of a painful episode and sometimes preceding it, these mostly take the form of moving spots, flashing lights, blurring or loss of vision (partial or, rarely, complete) rather than the hallucinatory images of the classic migraine. Hemianopia, teichopsia and fortification spectra do not emerge with any clarity, nor do hunger, euphoria, diarrhoea or polyuria appear to accompany cervical headaches. However, dysarthria, dysphasia, ataxia and loss of concentration sometimes do accompany a headache of cervical origin.

Depression, disorientation, paraesthesia (of face and extremities), hypogastric pain and globulus hystericus, although not common, have been recorded in association with headaches of cervical origin and have abated along with the pain after appropriate treatment of the cervical spine.

Attacks or episodes

When the patient describes the headache in terms of an attack it is more likely to be a migraine. A typical attack is described as follows. It may occur spontaneously or at a certain time after a known precipitating factor or at a certain time of the day or month or year. Frequently there is some foreknowledge that an attack is imminent and the patient knows what sequence of symptoms and progression of pain to expect. She also knows how long it will last. Nausea and vomiting usually accompany an attack, but are also common in severe cervical headaches. Once the pain is fully developed, the patient is prostrated and will, if possible, lie in a darkened room with a damp cloth on her forehead and remain there until the attack has passed. This may be hours or days. Commonly after an attack the patient is exhausted for a period, after which she is quite symptom-free until the next attack.

It is unusual for a cervical headache to occur in this manner. The headaches are not confined to attacks but fluctuate according to circumstances. As the lesion of the cervical spine progresses, the pain is more easily provoked by less potent precipitants. This results in an increase in the periodicity of pain, which at a certain stage becomes continuous. This factor typifies the cervical headache more reliably than any other.

Onset and course

These differ sufficiently to be diagnostic if clearly established. The onset of a migraine is usually related to puberty, and the pain/periodicity pattern established at its onset is more or less maintained through the years until it abates in later life.

The onset of the cervical headache is unrelated to puberty and may occur at any stage from infancy to old age depending on the onset of the cervical lesion. Frequently there is a late post-traumatic osteoarthrosis. The pain/periodicity pattern increases gradually over the years, or suddenly after trauma to the head or neck. There may be periods of remission but untreated it does not abate in time.

Aetiology

Some investigators believe that migraine is linked to childhood motion sickness and allergy and that there is a strong familial element. I have found these three factors to be present in so many cases of cervical headache that they cannot relate exclusively to migraine. The fact that cervical headaches so often occur in more than one member of a family is perhaps puzzling, but two possible reasons for this are (1) there may be a familial congenital anomaly in the cervical spine which predisposes to injury, or (2) the incidence of cervical headache in its various stages of development is so common that inevitably more than one member of many families are afflicted.

Diagnosis

The early cervical headache is readily diagnosed. It is well described by Brain (1963) but he does not make it clear that it is the early syndrome. The late post-traumatic fully developed cervical headache frequently eludes diagnosis because:

1. The initial injury (usually a blow to the head or a jolt to the neck many years before) has long been forgotten by the time the headache has become severe and frequent. This need not have been major trauma – it could have been repeated minor trauma or a congenital anomaly aggravated by unfavourable occupational head-on-neck positioning.
2. Radiological studies of the neck are usually unhelpful. Degenerative changes are commonly seen in X-rays of the neck which are unrelated to headache, and conversely, minor changes in the occipito-atlanto-axial joints, where the headache most often arises, are seldom demonstrable.
3. The confusion of symptoms suggests other diagnoses and leads to many unsuccessful treatments.
4. Neurological objective tests are negative.
5. Many of the traditional treatments for cervical spondylosis are ineffective because they are not accurately directed at the culprit structure.

Discussion

It is generally accepted that although cervicogenic headache and migraine constitute two separate pathological entities it is not uncommon for both to be operative in one subject. Careful questioning may elicit interwoven but typical histories of both.

It has not been conclusively established what it is that sets off the vasodilation of cranial blood vessels which results in migraine headache. Biochemical interactions, neurophysiological and psychological predisposition all play a role. There is speculation and study around the overt link between activity in the vertebral artery and upper cervical articular disorders; it seems that the close anatomical proximity of these structures makes it possible for a disorder in one to affect the other (Dutton and Riley, 1969).

Non-recurring headaches and other headaches which recur but are not common

The headaches referred to here will not be seen by the physical therapist but may not be ignored. Those therapists who become known as treaters of headache sometimes attract inappropriate cases and so we should know enough about 'other' headaches to be able to send them on to the right specialist.

Non-migrainous vascular

Headache associated with essential hypertension

Many people relate their headaches to their high blood pressure. However, hypertension has not been shown to be a cause of headache. Graham (1964) writes: 'There is a real question as to whether this headache should not be dealt with under the heading of "migraine" since there is much to suggest that the two are closely related.' Hypertensive patients who suffered headache were observed by Janeway (1913), Gardner *et al.* (1940) and Walker (1959) and it was found that they were the ones who previously were subject to migraine. Conversely, Graham argues if one follows migraine patients over many years, the emergence in them of hypertension and accentuation thereby of their migrainous headaches is surprisingly common. He goes on to say that these observations lead to the practical fact that measures directed against hypertension will help to prevent the accentuation of migraine which it promotes, and measures directed against migraine will help to quell the headache which hypertension has accentuated. Solomon (1991), however states that:

> 'several medications that are known to exacerbate migraine can also elevate blood pressure. These include amphetamines, cocaine, estrogens and oral contraceptives. Medications used in the treatment of hypertension can often exacerbate migraine. These include the vasodilators hydralazine, minoxidil, nifedipine, prazosin and reserpine. Several medications used in the treatment of hypertension are also effective in the prophylaxis of migraine.'

Another opinion (unpublished source) is that headaches are often experienced by patients who are aware of the fact that they are hypertensive and that these headaches start for the first time only after they become aware of the hypertension. Doctors often cause the patient to associate the two conditions because they believe that hypertension is responsible for headaches. Hypertension does apparently cause headache in a small number of cases but the great majority of patients with severe and malignant hypertension and who are unaware of it, do not experience headache. A sudden rise in blood pressure, especially in early benign hypertension, may cause headache but even if the blood pressure remains elevated the headache tends to disappear. It has the character of migraine but without the nausea and vomiting.

From the foregoing arguments it would seem reasonable to postulate that the anxiety occasioned by the diagnosis of hypertension could also result in sustained tension of the cervical muscles and render a quiescent cervical arthrosis symptomatic, causing headache.

Infection and inflammation

> 'The febrile response arising from inflammation in any part of the body may produce headache secondary to the cranial vasodilation which it creates. Headache due to this response must be separated from that arising from inflammation of cranial structures themselves. For example, influenza or brucellosis may cause headache owing to a generalized systemic toxic reaction, whereas cranial arteritis or encephalitis may create headache by direct implication of cranial structures. In any case, physical signs and laboratory findings suggesting the activity of an infectious or inflammatory process should alert the physician to the underlying disorder' (Graham, 1964).

Vascular headache associated with disorders of body chemistry and metabolism

> 'Headache due to cranial vasodilation not infrequently accompanies conditions in which hydration, electrolyte balance and body chemistry are disturbed. The dehydration commonly associated with febrile illness, especially if complicated by electrolyte loss due to vomiting and diarrhoea, prolongs and accentuates vascular headache until it is corrected by suitable replacement fluids given orally or parenterally. Since vomiting and diarrhoea may be an integral part of various headache syndromes, especially migraine, post-traumatic headache, and hypertensive encephalopathy, it is well to bear such replacement therapy in mind as well as the more specific measures directed at the aetiology of the original headache' (Graham, 1964).

Hypercapnia and anoxia, found in patients suffering severe pulmonary disease, create severe headache due to cranial vasodilation, at times associated with increased intracranial pressure and papilloedema. Proper ventilation is the treatment of choice. Vascular headache can be a symptom in many other conditions, e.g. cerebral hypoxia occurring during exposure to reduced oxygen tension at high altitudes or to the insidious presence of carbon monoxide, which explains the headache arising in stuffy rooms. Vascular headache usually complicates other sources of cerebral anoxia such as the sudden development of anaemia, whether by haemorrhage or haemolysis, cerebral artery obstruction from a clot, embolus or arteriosclerotic narrowing or kinking, or failure of the systemic circulation as in shock, postural hypotension or heartblock.

Vascular headaches due to chemical agents and foods

In this category are headaches produced by chemicals prescribed by physicians, sometimes as treatment for headache, e.g. reserpine (high dosage), Dexedrine, nitroglycerine, Apresoline, ephedrine, monoamine oxidase inhibitors, acetanilide, phenacetin, caffeine, various sedatives and corticosteroids. Histamine by injection may result in headache and insulin and oral antidiabetic agents may produce hypoglycaemic reactions of which vascular headache is a common symptom.

Caffeine may cause vascular headache in migrainous subjects. Too much coffee at the start of the day may lead to headache later on when its stimulation and vasoconstriction wear off, resulting in what is known as caffeine withdrawal headache. Alcohol frequently produces headache in migrainous subjects. This is common knowledge, but it is less well known that alcohol also can trigger the cervical headache (Edeling, 1982). Many liquors contain significant amounts of tyramine which in susceptible subjects, especially those under treatment with monoamine oxidase inhibitors, may produce severe pressor reactions and headache. Many patients report a tendency to get an attack of headache after eating chocolate. This may represent an allergic process, or the xanthine content of chocolate could act as a vasodilator.

Lumbar puncture headache

This headache has vascular components and relates to decreased volume of cerebrospinal fluid secondary to leakage through the needle hole in the spinal sac. The best therapy is for the patient to remain in such a position that the fluid no longer drains, that is with the foot of the bed raised for an hour after the procedure and then flat for a further eight hours.

The following is transcribed and quoted from Graham (1964) with some comment by the author:

> 'Tense patients may have a postpuncture headache of the muscle contraction or vascular variety such as may follow a period of anxiety related to any needling procedure.'

The author thinks that this is why we are sometimes able to relieve a post-lumbar puncture headache by means of mobilizing the cervical spine.

Miscellaneous cephalalgias (Rushton 1964)

Cranial arteritis

Cranial arteritis is accompanied by systemic symptoms of fatigue, weakness, anaemia, night sweats, weight loss, etc. and it requires early and vigorous medical treatment in order to prevent resulting blindness. Women and men over the age of 50 years who start headache for the first time should be suspect. The pain is uni- or bilateral and localized to the affected scalp arteries, but can be general. Pain in the jaw muscles while chewing may indicate intermittent claudication.

Objectively there is a tenderness and thickening of the temporal (or other scalp) arteries and they do not pulsate. The overlying skin could be inflamed. The erythrocyte sedimentation rate (ESR) is markedly increased but a normal ESR does not exclude the diagnosis. Histology of arterial biopsy is diagnostic, but as the lesions tend to be patchy a negative biopsy does not exclude the diagnosis. The treatment is medical.

Trigeminal neuralgia (tic douloureux)

This may occur in anyone over 50 years of age. Pain occurs in the distribution of the trigeminal nerve, usually the maxillary and mandibular divisions. There is sudden intense superficial shooting or stabbing pain which immobilizes the face – cheek, chin, lips and tongue. The patient may clutch his face. It is triggered by light skin touch like washing, shaving, and eating or talking. Attacks last less than a minute and there is no latent pain. There may be one or more paroxysms per day or repeated paroxysms every few seconds which may be perceived as continuous pain. Attacks may occur daily for weeks or months with remission of up to 24 months. Remission periods tend to shorten with the passage of time and the disease worsens. There are no clinical signs or sensory loss. The current treatment is medical with carbamazepine.

Post-herpetic neuralgia

Pain which persists more than eight weeks after the appearance of the vesicles may be referred to as post-herpetic neuralgia. It lasts for many months, slowly subsiding, often incompletely. The nerve most commonly involved in the head is the ophthalmic branch of the trigeminal. The pain varies from an annoying paraesthesia to sharp jabs of pain on a background of steady burning or aching. Many subjects become depressed. Medical and surgical treatment is disappointing and physiotherapy has nothing reliable to offer.

Atypical neuralgias
Sluder's neuralgia, vidian neuralgia, Charlin's syndrome, nasociliary neuralgia, petrosal neuralgia and migrainous neuralgia come under this heading. The common pain mechanism is abnormal vasodilation and no satisfactory treatment has yet been found.

Atypical face pain
This constitutes an ill-defined group which does not fall into any of the foregoing groups and where the pain cannot be shown to arise in the teeth, paranasal sinuses, eyes or ears. They should not go untreated and Rushton (1964) recommends simple analgesics, sedatives or tranquillizers and physiotherapy.

Disease of the temporomandibular joint
A distinction will need to be made between temporomandibular pain due to osteo- or rheumatoid arthritis and pain secondary to malocclusion and/or muscle hyperactivity of the temporalis muscle.

Many writers believe that the pain is primarily as a result of the muscle spasm and that treatment should be directed at relieving it. But it is true that the joint is often very tender to palpation and responds well to mobilization (*see* Chapter 10).

Headache in intracranial disorders

Headache is the initial symptom in 30% and is present in 80% of intracranial tumours. The headache is due to traction on pain-sensitive intracranial structures.

Sources of pain in intracranial disorders are:

1. Traction on intracranial blood vessels and venous sinuses.
2. Distention and dilation of intracranial blood vessels.
3. Inflammation in or about any pain-sensitive structures of the head.
4. Direct pressure by tumours on the cranial and cervical nerves containing many pain afferent fibres from the head.

> 'In contrast, the parenchyma of the brain, most of the dura and pia arachnoid, the ependymal layer of the ventricles, and the choroid plexuses are not pain-sensitive' (Bosches, 1964).

Subarachnoid haemorrhage
Headache resulting from subarachnoid haemorrhage involves sudden and dramatic onset of pain likened to a blow on the head. The pain is unilateral and rapidly becomes generalized, spreading to the back of the head and neck. There is a change in the level of consciousness and focal neurological signs and neck stiffness occur.

Meningitis and encephalitis
The onset of pain is usually over a period of hours or days but is sometimes sudden. It is bilateral, spreads down the neck and is aggravated by movement. There is photophobia, neck stiffness and fever.

Subdural haematoma
This almost always presents with a headache, usually accompanied by drowsiness. The onset is over a period of days or weeks, even in the absence of head injury.

Extradural haematoma
This is usually as a result of tearing of the middle meningeal artery at the site of a fracture and presents as an acute problem.

Headaches in children

Headache is not uncommon in children and because it can be a symptom of many disorders, all known cause of headache should be explored. Livingstone and Whitehouse (1964) discuss two of the disorders which give rise to recurring headaches in children, and these are epilepsy and migraine.

The reader should be aware that cervical headache also occurs in children and should be treated in the same way as in an adult, and that grade V manipulation should be avoided.

References

Bosches, B. (1964) Treatment of headache in intracranial disorders. In Friedman, A. P., ed., *Modern Treatment* (Symposium on the Treatment of Headache), Vol. 1, No. 6, pp. 1375–1383. Harper and Row, New York

Brain, R. (1963) Some unsolved problems of cervical spondylosis. *British Medical Journal*, **1**, 772

Chapman, S. (1986) A review and clinical perspective on the use of EMG and thermal biofeedback for chronic headaches. *Pain*, **24**, 1–43

Dutton, C. P. and Riley L. H. Jnr (1969) Cervical migraine: not merely a pain in the neck. *American Journal of Medicine*, **47**, 141–148

Edeling, J. (1974) Migraine and other chronic headaches. *South African Journal of Physiotherapy*, **36**, 13–17

Edeling, J. (1980) The subjective assessment of pain in orthopaedic joint problems *South African Journal of Physiotherapy*, **36**, 13–17

Edeling, J. (1982) The true cervical headache. *South African Medical Journal*, **62**, 531–534

Frazier, S. H. (1964) The psychotherapeutic approach to patients with headache. In Friedman, A. P., ed., *Modern Treatment* (Symposium on the Treatment of Headache), Vol. 1, No. 6, pp. 1412–1424. Harper and Row, New York

Gardner, J. W., Mountain, G. E. and Hines, E. A. (1940) The relationship of migraine to hypertension headaches. *American Journal of Medical Science*, **200**, 50

Graham, J. R. (1964) Treatment of non-migrainous vascular headache. In Friedman, A. P., ed., *Modern Treatment* (Symposium on the Treatment of Headache), Vol. 1, No. 6, pp. 1432–1440. Harper and Row, New York

Headache Classification Committee of the International Headache Society (1988) Classification and diagnostic criteria for headache disorders, cranial neuralgias and facial pain. *Cephalalgia. An International Journal of Headache*, **8**, (Suppl. 7)

Janeway, T. C. (1913) A clinical study of hypertensive cardiovascular disease. *Arch of Int. Med.*, **12**, 755

Jull, G. (1981) Clinical manifestations of cervical headache. In *Proceedings of a Symposium on Cervical Spine and Headache*, pp. 28–42. Manipulative Therapist's Association of Australia, Brisbane.

Kunkel, R. S. (1991) Diagnosis and treatment of muscle contraction (tension-type) headaches. *Medical Clinics of North America*, **75**, (3), 595–603

Livingstone, S. and Whitehouse, D. (1964) Treatment of headache in children. In Friedman, A. P. ed., *Modern Treatment* (Symposium on the Treatment of Headache), Vol. 1, No. 6. Harper and Row, New York

Pikof, H. (1984) Is the muscular model of headache still available? A review of conflicting data. *Headache*, **24**, 186–198

Rushton, J. G. (1964) Treatment of miscellaneous cephalalgias. In Friedman, A. P., ed., *Modern Treatment* (Symposium on the Treatment of Headache), Vol. 1, No. 6, pp. 1426–1431. Harper and Row, New York

Sjaastad, O. (1983) Cervicogenic headache. An hypothesis. *Cephalalgia*, **3**, 249–256

Solomon, G. D. (1991) Concomitant medical disease and headache. In Diamond, S., guest ed., *The Medical Clinics of North America. Headache* **75(3)**

Trevor-Jones, R. (1964) Osteo-arthritis of the paravertebral joints of the 2nd and 3rd cervical vertebrae as a cause of occipital headache. *South African Medical Journal*, **38**, 392–395

Walker, C. H. (1959) Migraine and its relationship to hypertension. *British Medical Journal*, 1430

Further reading

Borgeat, F., Hade, B., Elie R. and Larouche, C. M. (1984) Effects of voluntary muscle tension increases in tension headache. *Headache*, **24**, 199–202

Cohen, M. J. and McArthur, D. L. (1981) Classification of migraine and tension headache from a survey of 10,000 headache diaries. *Headache*, **21**, 25–29

Edeling, J. (1986) The abandoned headache syndrome. In Grieve, G. P., ed., *Modern Manual Therapy of the Vertebral Column*. Churchill Livingstone, Edinburgh

Edeling, J. (1980) Diagnosis by manipulation. in *Proceedings IFOMT 4th Conference* (Christchurch New Zealand). Eds Buswell, J, and Gibson Smith, M. Published with the assistance of the J. R. McKenzie Trust Board

Friedman, A. P. (1979) Characteristics of tension headache; profile of 1420 cases. *Psychosomatics*, **20**, 451–461

Haber J. D., Kuczmierczyk, A. R. and Adams H. (1985) Tension headaches: muscle overactivity or psychogenic pain. *Headache*, **25**, 23–29

Jay G. W. Brunson J. and Branson S. J. (1989) The effectiveness of physical therapy in the treatment of chronic daily headaches. *Headache*, **29**, 156–162

Kelgren, J. H. (1938) Observations on referred pain arising from muscle. *Clinical Science*, **3**, 175–190

Kelgren, J. H. (1939) On the distribution of referred pain arising from deep somatic structures with charts of segmental pain areas. *Clinical Science*, **4**, 35–46

Maxwell, H., ed. (1966) The diagnosis and differential diagnosis of headache. In *Migraine*, Ch. VII. John Wright and Sons, Bristol

Posniak, P. (1976) Cephalgic spasm of head and neck muscles. *Headache*, **15**, 261–266

Rocabado, M. (1983) Biochemical relationship of the cranial, cervical and hyoid regions. *Journal of Craniomandibular Practice. Physical Therapy*, **1**(3)

Rocabado, M. (1985) Arthrokinematics of the temporomandibular joint. In *Clinical Management of Head, Neck and TMJ pain and Dysfunction*. W. B. Saunders, London

Sutton, E. P. and Belar, C. D. (1982) Tension headache patients versus controls: a study of EMG parameters. *Headache*, **22**, 132–136

Thompson, J. K. and Adams H. E. (1984) Pathophysiological characteristics of headache patients. *Pain*, **18**, 41–52

3

Clinical differences between cervical headache and other vertebral pain

The chronic headache which arises from the craniovertebral and upper cervical joints (C1–C3) is a separate and unique symptom syndrome and needs to be clinically differentiated from disorders at other vertebral levels. The behaviour of the pain is quite different. Although this type of headache is very responsive to manipulative therapy, the methods of examination, assessment and treatment need to be substantially modified in order to reveal the true picture and to treat it with consistently good results.

The following comparison of clinical features should help the clinician gain a deeper insight into the condition of chronic cervical headache. The features belonging to complaints at other vertebral levels will be cited first, as these are more familiar.

Differences in subjective examination

The subjective examination for *other vertebral levels* is important, but much information may be gained from the physical examination. *Headache*, on the other hand, is a predominantly subjective complaint. There is more to be discovered from the patient's account of it than from physical tests. A wealth of information is available from the patient with chronic headache and because the presence of pain is such a constant feature, it is a very useful parameter for subjective assessment and reassessment. In order to make proper use of this information for reassessment, the subjective examination must be done in depth and from a basis of understanding of the headache syndrome as distinct from pain syndromes arising from other vertebral levels. The differences in the subjective perception of the chronic cervical headache pain and other vertebral pain syndromes follow.

Pain characteristic

When the patient describes *neckache* or *backache*, the nature of the local or referred vertebral pain is usually perceived to be either superficial or deep, burning, aching, dull or sharp, like toothache, or nauseating. The *headache* patient, however, more often describes some component of pressure, a throbbing or even a pounding pain. A feeling of inward or outwardly directed pressure as if the head is being crushed or is about to burst is common, as is the feeling of a tight band squeezing the head or of being pierced by a rod. Therapists and doctors who are not familiar with such florid descriptions are apt to think that the patient is overdramatizing her condition, but these perceptions are reported so consistently by headache sufferers that they must be genuine and do not indicate a neurotic patient.

Total pain pattern

Periodicity of pain

By periodicity is meant the frequency of the presence of pain. In the natural course of the syndrome through time, the presence of *neck*, *dorsal*, or *lumbar pain* tends to occur in irregular acute bouts, usually related to strain, initially self limiting and later requiring some form of treatment. In the case of *headache*, the pain, in the early stages of the syndrome, is infrequent and erratic. Over a period of time the headaches become more regular and ever more frequent, e.g. a once-a-month headache becomes a once-or twice-a-week headache, then daily, and finally continuous. It is not uncommon for a patient to have had a continuous headache for many years.

Intensity of pain

There are no marked differences here. *Other vertebral pain* and *headache* may reach alarming severity, but in the examination of headache, where the assessment is more heavily dependent on subjective information, it is useful to elicit and record the patient's estimate of pain intensity on a scale of 1–5, for purposes of reassessment. Patients are usually well able to perceive a lessening of pain intensity after the application of a trial therapeutic technique and this is very useful information for the therapist. It could also be helpful to know, for example, that a headache which had reached 4 on the intensity scale for at least two days a week, had not reached more than 2 in one week following the start of treatment.

Response to analgesics

No difference has been observed in this aspect between the two entities. At the higher levels of pain intensity the response to analgesics is poor, but it is useful to assess, initially, the current response to a certain dosage of analgesic. This serves two purposes in the case of *headaches*. One is to confirm the patient's estimate of the pain intensity, because the response to analgesics is roughly proportional to the level of pain. The other purpose is to help in the assessment of a decline in the syndrome. If a patient reports a better response to the same dosage or, if she needs analgesics less often than before, then the condition is improving.

Precipitating factors

There is a very marked difference between the conditions which bring on or aggravate a *backache* or *neckache* and those that bring on a *headache*. It is most important for the examiner to be aware of these differences. At all *other vertebral levels* the factors that trigger joint pain are predominantly mechanical and dynamic, the most common being positioning (sitting, etc.) and movement (bending, lifting, twisting).

In the case of *headache*, even though the pain derives from intervertebral joints there are other and more potent factors which exacerbate pain. The most prevalent of these is stress, which results in sustained contraction of cervical muscles. The sustained contraction, induced by mental anxiety or even, in an irritable condition, by minor irritation, compresses pressure-sensitive craniovertebral joints and results in headache. Unfavourable occupational postures frequently trigger headache but only if maintained for long periods, for example desk workers whose headaches become worse towards the end of the day. Furthermore, there are other triggers exclusive to the individual. These may include altitude, heat, glare, loud noise, driving in heavy traffic, smells, particular ingestants – in fact, anything which that individual headache sufferer finds personally irritating or offensive. It could be that these irritations also result in cervical muscle contraction.

Irritability

Irritability of a joint condition may be assessed by relating the behaviour of the symptoms to a particular function or activity. At *other vertebral levels* this usually involves certain movements which reproduce or aggravate the patient's pain. The more trivial the movement (e.g. lifting a shoe), the greater the pain evoked and the longer it lasts after the triggering movement has ceased, the more irritable the condition is judged to be.

As it is very seldom that a *headache* is evoked by a movement it is not possible to assess irritability in this way. A rough guide for headache irritability can be gained from the periodicity. The more frequently the headache occurs, e.g. daily or continuously, the more likely it is to be irritable. The fact that it is present so often means that it is constantly being triggered by trivia and does not spontaneously abate.

The condition causing headache at the craniovertebral joints is very likely to be irritable and to respond to initial disturbance from palpation with gross exacerbation of pain and other symptoms. Thus, it is wise to limit initial treatment to the barest minimum, as is suggested later in this text.

Associated symptoms

When examining *other vertebral joint conditions*, we seek certain symptoms in addition to pain. Nerve root involvement is suggested by the presence of paraesthesia, cutaneous anaesthesia and muscle weakness. We are on the look-out for cord involvement indicated by bilateral peripheral sensory disturbance, or for cauda equina pressure when there is bladder dysfunction and saddle anaesthesia. In the cervical spine, vertigo might indicate the compromise of the vertebrobasilar artery, to be differentiated from vestibular and other causes. Stiffness or a painful restriction of normal movement is also perceived subjectively by the patient. These symptoms suggest some complicating pathology and would influence the treatment approach.

In the case of *cervical headaches*, the associated symptoms are quite different and most do not indicate specific complicating pathology. Paraesthesia, muscle weakness and peripheral symptoms are rarely reported, nor are any of the other symptoms that go together with the other vertebral conditions, with the exception of dizziness, which is common with cervical headaches. Occasionally, the patient will say that her head feels too heavy for her neck: this is not due, I think, to muscle weakness but to a sense of discomfort due to the weight of the head on the pain source. When a headache patient reports a disturbance in gait, care should be taken to determine whether the ataxia is simply a result of disorientation due to severe pain or perhaps the effect of heavy medication, or whether it merits investigation by a neurologist.

The symptoms which accompany pain in chronic headache cases are legion and are not those expected to accompany other joint symptoms. They are often bizarre and therefore puzzling and frightening to the patient. She should be encouraged to describe them to the examiner, not because they indicate serious pathology, but to reassure her. They are part and parcel of the chronic headache syndrome, whether it is of migrainous or cervical origin and will ebb and flow with the severity of the pain. The patient should be told that these symptoms are very common in cases of chronic headache and that, although they may be unpleasant, she need not worry about their significance and that they will clear up when the headaches abate.

The most common associated symptoms are visual disturbances, usually blurred vision or flashing lights or spots moving before the eyes, tinnitus, dizziness, nausea and vomiting. Then there are many other strange symptoms. Some of these might alert the experienced therapist and suggest special investigations, and others will be recognized as being unusual but benign. It would, however, be responsible to report anything unfamiliar to the patient's medical doctor.

History

The history in the case of *other vertebral levels* is the basis for the diagnosis. It is not generally appreciated that the true *cervical headache syndrome* will also display a very typical and informative retrospective history. The following sequence of events is typical.

Onset

This may be at any age from extreme youth to advanced age.

Development of headache syndrome

Initially, the patient experiences infrequent mild to moderate headaches, unaccompanied by other symptoms. The patient thinks that these headaches are 'normal'. Analgesics are seldom necessary but are effective when taken.

The headaches become more frequent over the years until they are present most of the time. As the pain intensity and the frequency of headache increases, associated symptoms appear.

Previous trauma

Relevant trauma for *lumbar problems* involves flexion, lifting or torsion strains. The trauma is more immediate to the problem and the patient readily relates subsequent backache to the damage sustained by the back.

The patient seldom relates trauma to her *headache*, although careful questioning will more often than not reveal relevant trauma at some time before the onset or escalation of the headache. Relevant trauma could be a blow to or a fall onto the head, or a whiplash injury. Because the headaches usually begin a long time after the incident and because the development of the syndrome is insidious, the patient does not relate the two. Furthermore, the patient does not always know that headache can stem from the neck, whereas most people know that a leg pain can come from the back.

Previous treatment

In *other vertebral problems*, the diagnosis is usually readily made because physical tests and the more sophisticated testing procedures point the way and suitable treatment is soon instituted. When taking the history of the *cervical headache* patient, one soon becomes aware of numbers of specialist consultations, negative tests and failed treatment.

Differences in physical examination

Physiological movement testing

At *other vertebral levels*, e.g. the lumbar spine, physical signs are prominent. The patient moves in a guarded manner and physiological movement tests can be relied on to reveal measurable restriction commensurate with the severity of the pain. At the mid and lower cervical spine, neck and/or arm pain is easily reproduced by performing certain physiological movements of the neck. Such movements will be variably limited by pain and/or stiffness.

With *headache*, physiological movements of the neck often appear full range and pain free. Because the possible range of movement at 0–C1–C2 is very small, painful restrictions here may be overridden by movement at pain-free subjacent levels (White, 1978). Worth and Selvick (1986) write that routine examination of the craniovertebral joints should include: measurement in all planes; observation of unilateral bias during active movement; habitual postures; and compensatory mechanisms below these joints. Unless the examiner has exceptional skill and experience in the assessment of movement at upper cervical joints, loss of movement at these levels might not be detected at all. Therefore these movement signs would be of little clinical value for the purpose of identifying the lesion or of reassessment when trying to determine the response to trial treatment techniques. To a therapist or medical practitioner who is not skilled or experienced in such examination, the physiological movement aberration could go undetected and if he did not go on to examine the accessory movements, the neck could be excluded as the source of pain.

Accessory movement testing

At *other vertebral levels*, perception of restricted range of accessory movement is common and, because these joints are usually not as hypersensitive to the pressures used in testing, it is possible to perform a thorough movement palpation and determine the extent and direction of the restriction. In seeking the joint source of the *cervical headache*, as a result of the dominance of pain and pressure sensitivity of the headache-producing joints and because the condition is likely to be very irritable, it is wiser and more informative to assess the extent of the pain response and not the range of restriction of accessory movement.

The palpation tests for passive accessory intervertebral movement (PAIVM) for chronic headache should be severely limited in the early stages of examination. Due to their hypersensitivity, even the slightest pressure could set up an unacceptable exacerbation of symptoms. The joint which is responsible for the headache will be quickly and easily identified in most cases by its sharp pain response to Grade I pressure and often by the appropriate referral of pain to the head.

If the examination or early treatment procedures do not exacerbate the headache nor have the desired therapeutic effect, a full and analytical palpation test may be carried out in an attempt to extract more information.

Physical medical testing

Lesions at *other vertebral levels* are more readily demonstrated by means of X-rays, computed tomography (CT) scans, magnetic resonance imaging (MRI) screening, etc. The *headache* lesion in the upper cervical spine is seldom shown by means of such tests.

Differences in treatment

Technique

Whereas rotation, longitudinal or other indirect techniques are often the treatment of choice at *other vertebral levels*, they are not as consistently or immediately therapeutic for the relief of headache arising from craniovertebral levels. It is my experience that the treatment of choice is accurately localized direct thumb pressures used in the right direction on the side of pain.

Dosage

Dosage, defined as the product of the grade used and the number of *pressures* of that grade applied, should be carefully chosen. Dosages which would be acceptable and therapeutic at *other vertebral levels* are likely to exacerbate *headache* in an exaggerated manner. Grade I × 10 when used in the treatment of headache means 10 Grade I pressures and not ten volleys of 30 seconds of Grade I pressures, as may be used in treatment of other vertebral joints. Poor success in the treatment of headache is most commonly attributed to over-treatment. Exacerbation should be avoided by the initial use of not more than 5 Grade I pressures which, if accurately localized and directed, is often effective enough to immediately cause a headache not responding to complex analgesia to abate. In such a case it is equally true that if a stronger grade, e.g. Grade II had been used, or a Grade I pressure exerted ten or more times, there could be a bad flare-up of pain lasting for hours or days. Headaches are commonly over-treated in this way. Although such a reaction is useful because it has identified the lesion, the flare-up should be controlled.

Having identified a technique which relates directly to a pain in the head, it is best to use *only* that technique in the restrained manner suggested. Going on to mobilize several other possibilities for good measure leads to confusion when it comes to reassessment. One should try to get rid of the head pain by treating only the joints that have been identified as being the cause of it. Only if the headache repeatedly recurs or there is residual neck pain is it necessary to mobilize other painful joints. Some of these might well be subsymptomatic and to treat them unnecessarily could render them symptomatic.

References

Edeling, J. (1980) The subjective assessment of pain in orthopaedic joint problems. *South African Journal of Physiotherapy* **36**, 13–17

Maitland, G. D. (1986) *Vertebral Manipulation*, 5th edn. Butterworth, London

White, A. A. and Panjab, M. M. (1978) The clinical biomechanics of the occipitoatlantoaxoid complex. *Orthopaedic Clinics of North America*, **9**, 867–878

Worth, D. R. and Selvick, G. (1986) Movements of the craniovertebral joints. In *Modern Manual Therapy of the Vertebral Column*. Ed. Grieve, G. P. Churchill Livingstone, Edinburgh

4 Concepts

In this chapter, certain concepts basic to the understanding and effective use of the method taught in this book will be defined briefly and reference given to appropriate sources.

Cervical or cervicogenic headache

This headache has long been termed the 'cervical headache' but the preferred term is 'cervicogenic headache' (Sjaastad, 1983). Either term is used and refers to the same condition.

This is a non-vascular chronic headache; it is the headache which is a common feature of cervical disease or injury. The disease process may involve muscle, vascular or neural tissue but the primary source of the headache is to be found in the joints of the upper cervical spine. Pathological changes in these structures stimulate the adjacent end-organs, which register pain. Stimulation of these structures may refer pain to the head, which is perceived as headache.

The most common pathological painful disease of the neck which can give rise to headache is, in the clinical experience of the author, cervical spondylosis. Although the pain mechanism remains unclear, treatment directed at the painful hypomobility of the upper cervical spinal joints usually relieves the head pain. The upper cervical joints are within the receptive field of the trigeminocervical nucleus and thus have direct access to the neuro-anatomical pathways that mediate referred pain to the head (Bogduk, 1986).

Referred pain

Kelgren (1938, 1939) demonstrated and determined segmental pain referral patterns by injecting a saline solution at each segment and recording the area in which the pain was felt. Many workers in the orthopaedic field have described the phenomenon. It is well set out in the anatomy manuals of Romanes and Cunningham (1978) and Last (1960). Taylor *et al.* (1984) put forward possible bases for referred pain, and Bogduk (1986) wrote as follows:

> 'The anatomical substrate for referred pain is the convergence of afferents from one region of the body onto neurons in the CNS that also receive afferents from topographically separate regions. The trigeminocervical nucleus

provides a suitable location for this to occur in the case of head and neck pain. If units in the trigeminocervical nucleus that otherwise innervate the back of the head also received afferents from the cervical vertebral column, then noxious vertebral stimuli could cause pain to be perceived as arising from the back of the head. Alternatively, if units that received trigeminal afferents also received vertebral afferents, then pain in the forehead could be generated by noxious stimuli in the vertebral column.'

It has been demonstrated by clinical experiments in man that experimental painful stimuli in the upper neck produce referred pain in the head. From this fact we may deduce that pathologically painful lesions of any of the structures innervated by the upper cervical nerves are capable of producing pain which is referred to the head. These structures are: the receptive field of the upper three cervical nerves, which includes the joints and ligaments of the upper three cervical segments; their posterior and anterior muscles; the sternocleidomastoid and trapezius muscles; the dura mater of the posterior cranial fossa; and the vertebral artery.

'The C1 spinal nerve has frequently been misrepresented as having no sensory distribution, but this erroneous view refers to the fact that usually it has no specific cutaneous branch. It is, nevertheless, sensory to deep suboccipital tissues. The C1 dorsal ramus supplies the suboccipital muscles. The C1 ventral ramus supplies the atlanto-occipital joint, . . .' (Bogduk, 1986).

Trauma and headache

Trauma is a very common cause of chronic headache. In the 1988 publication of the Headache Classification Committee of the International Headache Society, Section 5.2 describes diagnostic criteria for 'chronic post-traumatic headache', but features only the effects of head trauma on intracranial tissue. The headache which arises from intracranial injury is usually self limiting. It is the headache which stems from injury to the craniocervical joints which leads to the worsening chronic cervicogenic headache syndrome and accounts for a large proportion of the headaches treated by manipulative therapists.

Brain (1973) wrote:

'There may be more than one factor in the causation of headache following head injury. Although it might be expected that chronic changes within the skull, for example, meningeal adhesions, would play an important part in causing headache after head injury, similar headaches are rare after operations on the brain and meninges. Extracranial structures may therefore be an important source of headache, especially the muscles and joints of the upper part of the neck and upper cervical sensory nerves.'

In similar vein, Cyriax (1984), when discussing post-concussion headache, wrote: 'Naturally any force severe enough to cause concussion must expend some of its impact on the neck as well.'

It is usual for headaches following head or neck trauma to begin a long time after the injury. Initially, the headaches occur infrequently and are mild; this reflects the early syndrome, which typically worsens over the years to become the severe condition of the late post-traumatic cervical headache syndrome (described in the cervical headache profile in Chapter 2).

Migraine

The source of pain in migraine is to be found in the intra- and extracranial blood vessels. The blood vessel walls are pain sensitive to distension, traction or displacement. The idiopathic dilation of cranial blood vessels, together with an increase in a pain-threshold-lowering substance, result in headache for the migraine sufferer. Wolff (1963) theorized that a sterile inflammation occurs in addition to the vasodilation, that this inflammation is induced, neurogenically, by a neurokinin and a proteolytic enzyme, and that a transudation of fluid into cranial tissue occurs during a migraine attack.

Appenzeller (1991) reviews briefly the opinions held over the past 50 years about the aetiology of migraine. He discusses currently acceptable theories which include: a hypothesis of cerebral hypoxia; neuronal theories that the brain is the primary and initiating organ responsible for migraine attacks and the vascular pathogenesis; and an additional cellular theory of causation that attributes migraine attacks to dysfunction of endothelial cells.

The Headache Classification Committee of the International Headache Society (1988), has discarded the former terms *classical migraine* and *non-classical migraine* in favour of *migraine with aura* and *migraine without aura*. In migraine with aura there are focal neurological symptoms which localize to the cerebral cortex or brainstem. The aura is now the preferred term for what was known as the prodrome. Migraine without aura was known as common migraine.

Migraine has many variants and diagnostic criteria are supplied by the Classification. However, as diagnostic criteria for all headache forms overlap to a considerable extent, a differential diagnosis is offered in Chapter 2. For our purposes this will enable the therapist, by skilful questioning, to distinguish the vascular from the cervicogenic headache (or *tension headache* as it is thought of by the medical experts).

Treatment is by means of medically prescribed drugs and is aimed at reversing the vasodilation. Some are prescribed for symptomatic relief and others for ongoing prophylactic management. The patient's doctor is responsible for this treatment. The treatment as described in this book will not relieve migraine. (Friedman, 1979; Appenzeller, 1991; Diamond, 1991). When cervical manipulation *does* relieve a migraine, it suggests either that the migraine had a cervical component or that the cervical headache only resembled a migraine. The final diagnostic criterion should be a trial by cervical manipulation (Edeling, 1980).

Tension headache

Nearly all the diagnostic criteria for tension-type headache put forward over the years and published in the 1988 Classification could equally apply to cervical headache and indeed, to migraine. In the experience of the author those headaches which are diagnosed medically as 'tension' headaches respond readily to mobilization of joints and poorly to massage of muscles. The reader should examine, assess and treat tension headaches in the way to be described in this book because, although scalp and cervical muscle tension plays an important role in the exacerbation of cervicogenic headache, it is a trigger and not the primary cause of the pain (*see* Introduction to the second edition).

Combined headache

The vascular migraine and the cervicogenic headache, alias tension headache, may be present in the same subject and should be distinguished and treated accordingly (*see* Chapter 2); it is transcribed for the patient in Chapter 5. Many studies have been carried out to examine the overt relationship between migraine and cervical/tension headaches and many opinions proffered and rejected (*see* Bogduk, 1986). Irritation of the vertebral nerve by arthritis of the cervical spine was a theory supported by many authors. It has been stated that irritation of the vertebral nerve by cervical disc and other lesions produces an autonomic barrage which results in spasm of the vertebrobasilar system; this produces head pain by causing ischaemia of the vessel walls (Pawl, 1977). This theory is attractive but is not supported by recent studies. It has been shown, however, that the vertebral artery has a sensory innervation, via the vertebral nerve, from the C1, C2 dorsal roots (Kimmel, 1960). Thus the vertebral artery is a potential source of cervical headache.

Treatment of pain by passive movement

Although it is not known for certain how and why manipulation works, Wells *et al.* (1988) have supplied a concise rationale for the pain relief and other effects of manipulative procedures directed at spinal and peripheral joints. The aims of this treatment are given as:

1. decreasing pain and other symptoms
2. decreasing muscle spasm
3. improving mobility of the joints and soft tissues.

The mechanism whereby these effects are achieved by treatment is probably one or more of the following:

1. An alteration in the bias of sensory input from joints and soft tissues by an increase in stimulation of the mechanoreceptors located within them (Gate Control Theory: Melzack and Wall, 1965).
2. Reflex effects on spasm.

3. Prevention or limitation of the formation of inelastic scar tissue and restoration of extensibility to the soft tissues.
4. Improvement of tissue – fluid exchange.
5. Psychological effects of being carefully assessed and treated sympathetically.

In the assessment of cervical headache, the prompt abatement of head pain following judicious passive movement of the joints responsible for the pain confirms the clinical fact of pain relief by passive movement, thus leaving it for the researchers to find the exact neuro-anatomical pathogenesis.

Selection of techniques by a process of ongoing assessment

In essence, the method of Maitland (1986) of treating joint symptoms involves:

1. Locating and evaluating the offending joint by means of thorough subjective and physical examination.
2. Assessing the relevant signs and symptoms prevailing before the application of a technique.
3. Applying a trial technique.
4. Reassessing the signs and symptoms.
5. If there is an improvement, that technique is used until maximum advantage has been gained by its use. If no improvement is assessed after the application of the technique, it should be discarded and another evaluated in the same way.

Physiological and accessory movement

Physiological movement is that which can be carried out voluntarily by the patient, e.g. flexion and extension of the cervical column. But in every joint there is a degree of movement which cannot be voluntarily achieved. It is a certain extent of 'joint play' which is essential to normal joint function and the movement can only be produced by means of an extraneous force such as the hands of the manipulator. This is called accessory movement.

For example, in an interphalangeal joint the physiological movement is flexion and extension whereas accessory movement of rotation, side flexion, antero-posterior and postero-anterior movement, lateral glide, compression and distraction may be produced by the therapist. These accessory movements can also be produced by the therapist in the intervertebral joints. Accessory movement also implies that movement which lies beyond the voluntary range of a physiological movement and can only be obtained by the therapist exerting overpressure at the end of the range.

Manipulation and mobilization

Manipulation implies that the therapist, using his hands, moves the joint or joints to be manipulated to the end of the physiological or accessory range and there imparts a short amplitude, high velocity thrust. The intention is to free the joint of restrictive elements which limit the normal range. But, whereas this technique is the treatment of choice in certain joint conditions, it is not ideal for all. In some cases, for example where there is loss of patency of a vertebral artery, it would be contraindicated.

Movement in painful and stiff joints can be restored in a more gently persuasive manner by imparting oscillating passive movement. There are few conditions for which this technique would be contraindicated. It is known as 'mobilization' and is described by Maitland (1986) and forms the basis of the treatment advocated in this textbook.

Symptomatic, subsymptomatic and asymptomatic

When the patient is aware of pain or other symptoms arising from a joint (or other source), that joint may be said to be symptomatic, for example an arthrotic atlanto-axial joint which is painful to the extent that the patient is aware of pain, whether local or referred.

The same lesion may, however, be present but not subjectively perceived. On examination there will be signs of joint abnormality but the patient is not aware of it. Such a joint could be said to be subsymptomatic.

When treating a symptomatic cervical lesion which, in the context of this textbook presents as headache, the aim of the treatment is not to cure the condition as the arthrosis cannot be reversed. The aim is rather to restore the joint to a subsymptomatic state, in which state it may have been for years prior to the onset of symptoms. The chronic headache syndrome, which had been escalating over the years as the joint function worsened, abates. Because the underlying abnormality remains it will always be a potentially symptomatic joint under unfavourable conditions, but the symptom syndrome need never again escalate once it has responded to a regimen of mobilization of the culpable joint or joints. The aim of mobilization is to restore the joint condition to the subsymptomatic state.

An asymptomatic joint is one from which no symptoms arise because there is no potentially symptomatic abnormality. Maitland calls this a normal joint. All its movements, physiological and accessory, will be found to be of full and pain-free range.

Localized and regional manipulation

Manipulation is a short amplitude, high velocity, controlled passive movement carried out at the end of the physiological or accessory range of movement. When using such technique for spinal conditions, most manipulators apply the manipulation to the vertebral region which contains the lesion, e.g. rotation of the lumbar or cervical spine. This is a Grade V technique and is referred to as a regional manipulation. It would be recorded by Maitland as, for example, lumbar rotation to the left, Grade V.

In certain conditions where it is appropriate, Maitland localizes the thrust as closely as is possible to one or two intervertebral levels and calls this a localized manipulation. The symbol to indicate this technique is l/V (localized grade V) for example, left rotation, C1/2 l/V.

Stress in relation to cervicogenic headache

The painful pathology of the suboccipital structures causes a physiological muscle spasm which is splinting and protective in intent. Psychologically-induced muscle tension, when evoked, is added to the physiologically-induced tension and the resultant cumulative pressure is brought to bear on the already painful structures, particularly the pressure-sensitive disorder of the articular tissue and this greatly increases the pain of the headache. Stress and resultant muscle tension constitute a potent trigger for cervicogenic headache. In the early cervical headache syndrome it takes a lot of stress to evoke a headache but in the fully developed syndrome the minor irritations of daily living are sufficient to trigger the headache. This is because of the increased irritability of the advanced condition. This irritability decreases and abates with mobilization therapy and the patient reverts to the situation of the early syndrome when stress was not such a potent trigger.

Osteoarthrosis in relation to chronic headache

Painful hypomobility of cervical apophyseal or central joints can be palpated in most cases of chronic headache and usually proves to be the source of the referred head pain. If this is so, mobilization of the stiff joints relieves the pain. Osteoarthrosis may or may not be seen on X-ray and if seen, is not always discernable at the joint at which the pain source is palpated. This might be because the soft tissues are painful before bony changes are visible. Whatever the reason, the negative radiological findings too often preclude the correct diagnosis of cervical headache or treatment, and sometimes invasive treatment such as surgery is directed at the wrong structure.

The patient's history will suggest one of the causes of the osteoarthrosis or spondylosis. The ageing process, past craniocervical trauma and the long-term effects of postural imbalance all play an important role in the development of the arthrotic condition.

Posture in relation to headache

The long-term result of postural deformity may be a causative factor in the development of osteoarthrosis and chronic cervical headache. Janda (1987) describes a typical muscle imbalance syndrome and calls it the 'proximal or shoulder crossed syndrome'. In standing there is elevation and protraction of the shoulders as well as rotation and abduction of the scapulae, some winging of the scapulae and a forward head posture. The pectorals, upper trapezius, levator scapulae and sternocleidomastoid muscles have become tight. The craniomandibular muscles as well as the small muscles connecting the occiput and the cervical spine also tend to become tight and the lower stabilizers of the scapulae become weakened and inhibited. This abnormal posture stresses the cervicocranial and cervicothoracic junctions and also the craniomandibular joint.

Rocabado (1993 personal communication) describes development of the same postural deformity which eventually results in osteoarthrosis of the cervical spine. According to his observations it often begins in childhood with a mouth breather. Mouth breathers adopt a 'head forward' posture which allows a posterior rotation of the cranium on the cervical spine, closing down the suboccipital space. The alignment of the cervical spine adapts. The normal lordosis flattens and in time becomes inverted. The anterior aspects of the vertebral bodies impact and erode and there is a posterior thrust. Osteoarthrosis eventually develops with resultant head and neck pain.

Rocabado (1983) analysed the craniovertebral relationship, position of the hyoid bone and curvatures of the cervical spine showing a method of cephalometric tracing which relates the cranium, cervical spine, mandible and hyoid bone in a biomechanical functional unit. These relationships can be modified through manual orthopaedic techniques, or through removable orthopaedic appliances and he suggests that these two approaches should be clinically coordinated in order to re-establish the normal orthostatic position of the head on the neck and the normal craniomandibular relationship. It is suggested that an uncorrected faulty relationship of these structures leads to early joint degeneration.

Posture is also a trigger factor for chronic headache. Sustained unfavourable postures will often bring on or aggravate a headache. It is one of the factors which must be addressed in cases which respond incompletely to mobilization (*see* Chapter 14).

Muscle spasm as a primary source of pain

Cyriax (1975) writes, when referring to orthopaedic painful conditions:

> 'Muscle spasm is a secondary phenomenon and its treatment should be that of the primary disorder. The notion of ''fibrositis'', with its emphasis on alleged primary disease of muscle, has led to ... misconceptions. One is painful muscle spasm fixing a joint. The spasm is thought to be primary, but it is

merely called into being by a protective reflex originating elsewhere. Capener (1966) has lent his authority to the idea of painful muscle spasm in "acute derangements of the lower spine". In his view, the muscle spasm overshadows everything else and as soon as it is controlled the trouble begins to subside. The converse is the case, as can be proved by epidural local anaesthesia which cannot reach the lumbar muscles. When the disc displacement recedes, the pain, felt in the muscles but not originating in them, and muscle guarding abate together. In orthopaedic disorders, the muscle spasm is secondary and is the result of, not the cause of pain; it causes no symptoms of itself. It is only cramp and neurogenic spasm that hurt muscles. Muscle spasm is thought to require treatment, as evidenced by the many muscle relaxants that are advertised for the cure of lumbago, for example. Osteopaths attribute all sorts of dire diseases to vertebral muscle spasm. The treatment of muscle spasm is of the lesion to which it is secondary; it never of itself requires treatment in lesions of the moving parts. . . . Spasm is thus the reaction, indeed the only reaction of which a contractile structure is capable, to any lesion of sufficient severity in its neighbourhood.'

This concept is basic to Maitland's approach and is accepted and used to good effect by manipulative therapists (Maitland, 1986).

References

Appenzeller, O. (1991) Pathogenesis of migraine. In Diamond, S., guest ed., *Medical Clinics of North America*, **75** (3) 763–791.

Bogduk, N. (1986) Cervical causes of headache and dizziness. In Grieve, G. P., ed., *Modern Manual Therapy of the Vertebral Column*. Churchill Livingstone, Edinburgh

Brain W. R. (1973) *Brain's Clinical Neurology* revised by Roger Bannister. Oxford University Press, Oxford

Capener, N. (1966) Vulnerability of the posterior interosseus nerve. *Journal of Bone and Joint Surgery*, **48B**, 770

Cyriax, J. (1975) Muscle spasm. Referred pain. In *Textbook of Orthopaedic Medicine, Vol. 1, Diagnosis of Soft Tissue Lesions*, 6th edn., pp. 9–13, 28–30, Baillière and Tindall, London

Cyriax, J., ed. (1984) Diagnosis of soft tissue lesions. In *Textbook of Orthopaedic Medicine*, 6th edn. Baillière and Tindall, London

Diamond, S., ed. (1991) Migraine headaches. *Medical Clinics of North America*, **75** (3) 545–566

Edeling, J. (1980) Diagnosis by manipulation. In *Proceedings IFOMT 4th Conference* (Christchurch, New Zealand), Eds Buswell, J. and Gibson Smith, M. Published with the assistance of the J. R. McKenzie Trust Board

Friedman, A. P. (1979) Characteristics of tension headache: a profile of 1,420 cases. *Psychosomatics*, **20**, 451–461

Headache Classification Committee of the International Headache Society (1988). Classification and diagnostic criteria for headache disorders, cranial neuralgias and facial pain. *Cephalalgia. An International Journal of Headache*, **8** (Suppl. 7)

Janda, V. (1987) Muscles and cervicogenic pain syndromes. In Grant, R., ed., *Clinics in Physical Therapy, Physical Therapy of the Cervical and Thoracic Spine* Vol. 1, (17) 153–166. Longman, London

Kelgren, J. H. (1938) Observations on referred pain arising from muscle. *Clinical Science*, **3**, 175–190

Kelgren, J. H. (1939) On the distribution of referred pain arising from deep somatic structures with charts of segmental pain areas. *Clinical Science*, **4**, 35–46

Kimmel, D. L. (1960) Innervation of the spinal dura mater and dura mater of the posterior cranial fossa. *Neurology*, **10**, 800–809

Last, R. J. (1960) *Anatomy – Regional and Applied*: J. and A. Churchill, Edinburgh

Maitland, G. D. (1986) *Vertebral Manipulation*, 5th edn., pp. 175–176. Butterworths, London

Melzack, R. and Wall, P. D. (1965) Pain mechanism: a new theory. *Science*, **150**, 971–979

Pawl, R. P. (1977) Headache, cervical spondylosis and anterior cervical fusion. *Surgical Annual*, **9**, 391–408

Rocabado, M. (1983) Biomechanical relationship of the cranial, cervical and hyoid regions. *Journal of Craniomandibular Practice. Physical Therapy*, **1** (3) 61–66

Romanes, G. J. and Cunningham, D. J., eds. (1978) Head and neck pain. In *Romanes Manual of Practical Anatomy*, 14th edn. Oxford University Press, New York

Sjaastad, O. (1983) Cervicogenic headache. An hypothesis. *Cephalalgia*, **3**, 249–256

Taylor D. C. M., Pierau, Fr-K., Mizutani, M. (1984) Possible bases for referred pain. In Holden A. V. and Winlow, W., eds., *The Neurobiology of Pain* pp. 143–56. Manchester University Press, Manchester

Wells, P. E., Frampton, V. and Bowsher D., eds. (1988) In *Pain. Management and Control in Physiotherapy*. Butterworth-Heinemann, Oxford

Wolff H. G., eds. (1963) In *Headache and Other Head Pain*, 2nd edn., Oxford University Press, New York

Further reading

Brain, W. R. (1954) Cervical spondylosis. *Lancet*, **i**, 687

Brain, W. R. (1963) Some unsolved problems of cervical spondylosis. *Brritish Medical Journal.*, **1**, 772

Jull, G. (1978) Clinical observations of upper Cervical Mobility. Proc. of Inaugural Congress of the MTAA Sydney

Jull G. (1981) Clinical Manifestations of Cervical Headache. In: Proc. Symp Cervical Spine and Headache. Brisbane Manipulative Therapist's Association of Australia; 28–42

Lance J. W.(1973) Mechanism and Management of Headaches. Butterworth-Heinemann, Oxford

Watson J. (1986) Pain and Nociception- Mechanisms and Modulation. In Grieve, G. P., ed., *Modern Manual Therapy of the Vertebral Column*. Churchill Livingstone. Edinburgh

5 Concepts transcribed for the patient

In this chapter certain concepts which will help the patient to understand her headache condition are presented in a simplified narrative. This information should be offered on a selective basis. Some patients simply wish to be rid of their pain and if it abates from passive treatment they are content. Others show an intellectual interest in the condition and wish to learn more about it. Those who do not respond well to treatment will need to take an informed part in the ongoing management of the condition and guidelines for this are given in Chapter 14.

At the first visit or soon after most patients will want to know what is causing the headache. They will have had numerous tests which did not reveal the cause. They fear covert malignant intracranial pathology. Many will have been diagnosed as tension headaches or migraine but medical treatment for these conditions has been ineffective and they want to know how physical treatment can help them. It is important for them to gain insight and understanding of the condition which plagues them. It would be wise to offer the explanation *after* the initial assessment has been made.

Before understanding the cervical headache the patient will need to know about pain referral. Many patients will be aware of the fact that pain felt in one part of the body could be coming from another and are content with this brief statement of fact. But others will want to know 'how that works'. A simplified narrative follows.

How pain is referred

When the foetus develops in the uterus, its length is organized into segments which will correspond with those of the spinal cord and vertebrae. From each segment a 'slice' of the body develops. In each segmental slice a portion of skin, muscle, bone and the internal organs (viscera) develops. At each segment nerves develop which will serve the skin and the deeper tissues contained in that 'slice'. Those nerves that serve deep structures and those that serve superficial structures in each slice enter and exit the spinal cord at the same point. Because this is so, there is a shared pathway from that point up to the sensory cortex of the brain and the brain is not always able to distinguish whether the message comes from the skin or from a deeper structure within that segment, for example, a joint.

Thus, the nerves which convey feeling (e.g. pain) to the brain from a deep structure such as an intervertebral joint enter the spinal cord at the same level as those which convey feeling from the portion of skin, muscle or bone which developed from the same segment as that particular joint. Thus the brain easily mistakes the source of that pain and interprets it as coming from the corresponding more superficial area of skin, muscle or bone. For example, if there is pain in the 5th cervical intervertebral joint (C5) the brain could think that the pain is coming from the portion of the arm which developed from the 5th cervical segment. The patient could have severe pain in her arm when there is nothing *in* the arm which is causing pain. In the case of cervical headache, there is nothing *in* the head which is causing the pain. The pain is in the upper joints of the neck but feels as if it is somewhere in the head.

The cervical headache

There are many different causes of headache. Almost everyone will have had a headache at some time or other but they will not all require specific treatment. A pain pill will usually suffice. Headaches are but one of the symptoms of many diseases, e.g. influenza. But when the 'flu has abated the headache will also have gone. Such headaches are called non-recurring headaches.

There are also recurring or chronic headaches, and these seems to be your (the patient's) problem. Chronic headaches occur in the absence of any discernable disease. They occur regularly over a period of many years and nothing seems to help them. There are mainly two causes of chronic headache. One is 'migraine', which one often hears or reads about. The other is the cervical headache which comes from the intervertebral joints of the neck. It is better known as tension headache because it is so much influenced by muscle tension of the neck muscles. This what you (the patient) probably have and if it is, then this treatment will help.

The pain that you feel in your head isn't inside your head but in your neck. The vertebral joints where your head joins your neck have become extremely painful, but you are not always aware of neck pain and it feels to you that the pain is in the head. In the same way, pain in the vertebrae of the lower back is often felt in the leg and called sciatica. But the pain is not in the leg, it is in the back. This is a well-known phenomenon and is called *referred pain* (*see* above).

The painful condition in these joints is commonly called osteoarthritis but the more correct term is osteoarthrosis. This condition must not be confused with rheumatoid arthritis. Rheumatoid arthritis is an inflammatory disease that attacks joints and destroys them. Osteoarthrosis is not so much a disease as a process of wear and tear and is a mechanical rather than an inflammatory disorder. The joint surfaces become eroded and rough with the result that the joint becomes stiff.

Now the only function of a joint is that of movement. When a joint becomes stiff and can no longer move as it should it is a sick joint and becomes very painful. It is actually the *stiffness* that results in pain and not the osteoarthrosis itself. Many joints which show signs of osteoarthrosis on X-ray studies are not painful. And so it follows that if we are able to relieve the stiffness the pain will abate. The treatment you (the patient) will receive for your headache is called 'mobilization' and is based on this principle. Mobilization involves your therapist imparting very gentle oscillating pressures to the joint which is responsible for the pain. This is to loosen up the stiffness and it is very effective in restoring the arthrotic joints to their previously subsymptomatic state (*see* Chapter 4).

The causes of osteoarthrosis are many. One of these is simply the wearing down of the joint surfaces of weight-bearing joints over a period of many years. This is why osteoarthrosis is so common in elderly people.

However, many young people suffer from osteoarthrosis which can arise from a variety of conditions, e.g. meningitis, which is an inflammation of the covering of the brain and spinal cord. These conditions involve the joint structures being attacked, leaving them stiff indefinitely after the inflammatory stage has subsided. Other relevant inflammatory conditions include Scheuermann's disease and rheumatic fever. Mechanical causes include congenital malalignment of intervertebral joints and/or postural imbalance caused, for instance, by old polio or other causes of muscle weakness; the osteoarthrosis results from sustained abnormal strains imposed on the joint structures.

Another very common cause of osteoarthrosis is an injury in the past which has damaged the fragile joint structures. The healing process of ligaments and cartilage often results in the formation of pain-sensitive scar tissue which restricts the movement of the joint. This process goes on for a very long time causing the joint to become ever more stiff and painful through the years. In the case of the headache which arises in the damaged skull–neck joints, the headaches often begin many years after the injury. At first, there is only minor stiffness, but as the stiffness progresses the joint becomes more and more painful and the headaches more frequent. This is why the cervical headache condition typically worsens over the years. Usually it is only when the headache becomes frequent and more severe that the patient will seek treatment. Before this stage it is often thought to be normal to have headaches from time to time. But it doesn't matter if it is left until this late stage before commencing treatment. Loosening the stiff joints, even at an advanced stage of degeneration, can free them of the pain.

If your headache has a purely mechanical cause, it can be expected to respond quickly and completely to treatment by joint mobilization. The headaches should cease to be a problem. However, other pathology sometimes complicates the response to treatment, the joints respond incompletely and the headaches persistently recur. If this should be so in your case your therapist will explore the other possibilities and will expect you to take a more active part in the management of the condition (*see* Chapter 14)

Tension headache

'Tension headache' is really just another name for 'cervical headache'. Although tension plays a large role in the cervical headache, it is not the *cause*.

Tension of the neck muscles acts on the painful underlying joints making them even more painful and the headache ensues (*see* Stress section below).

Migraine

Migraine is a chronic headache condition but the source of the pain is not in the neck joints and, of course, treating these joints cannot help it. Migraine is a 'vascular' headache, which means that the pain comes from the blood vessels of the head. In migraine sufferers the walls of these blood vessels dilate from time to time. When these blood vessels are stretched in this way they hurt and it is thought that this is what causes the pain of vascular headaches or migraine.

It is not known exactly what causes this dilation, and the treatment of migraine involves drugs which act on the blood vessels and cause them to constrict and return to their normal diameter, allowing the pain to subside. In some cases prophylactic drugs are given on a permanent basis in order to prevent attacks. If you suffer from migraine your medical doctor will advise you and prescribe the correct drug for you. There are many variants of migraine and the drug must be prescribed specifically for yours.

Combined headache

Sometimes the cervical headache and the migraine are both present in the same person. You may be aware of the fact that you have two different sorts of headache, for example one which is there very often (the cervical headache) and another which is seldom but is *different* (the migraine). It is possible for your therapist to distinguish between these two headaches (*see* Chapter 2). When a cervical headache condition is superimposed on that of migraine the migraine often becomes more frequent. The patient should be treated for the cervical headache and the expectations of this treatment are that the frequent cervical headache should clear up and that the migraine will revert to its former low frequency. Appropriate medication should be prescribed for the vascular migraine.

How stress affects headache

When an animal or a human is subjected to a stressful situation, for example when threatened, the muscles of the neck and shoulder girdle automatically contract in order to deal with the crisis. If physical action ensues and those tensed muscles are used to combat the threat, either by a fight or by fleeing from the danger, the energy will have been spent and those muscles will return to the previous relaxed state. If no physical action ensues, the muscles will relax, but over a longer period and incompletely.

If stressful incidents occur every day and even several times in one day, complete relaxation is not reached before the next irritation occurs. Thus, these muscles are almost never relaxed. Even when the person goes to sleep these muscles do not automatically let go. The day's anxieties are carried into the night and this person will wake the next morning tired and disgruntled after a very unsatisfactory night's rest. In this way the tension in the neck becomes a sustained muscle contraction. The muscles in themselves start to ache, but it is the sustained pressure that the tight muscles exert on the painful cranio-vertebral joints that triggers or aggravates the headache. These joints are exceptionally intolerant of even brief and slight pressure.

The patient often volunteers that her headache comes on or gets worse when she is under stress. This may be an accumulated effect of sustained stress such as anxiety or an acute incident like an angry confrontation. (For practical self help *see* Chapter 14.)

6

Factors that can trigger joint pain

In the presence of a lesion other than in the neck, the following factors can make any subsymptomatic joint symptomatic:

1. Unfavourable positioning, e.g. a patient with an osteoarthritic knee who is obliged to work in a squatting position or one with a lumbar problem sitting in a deep armchair.
2. Pressure. A swollen ankle is not necessarily painful unless there is an underlying joint lesion upon which the oedema is exerting pressure. Much of the joint pain can be relieved by getting rid of the oedema. Similarly premenstrual fluid retention can render a quiescent lumbar lesion painful. The pressure factor is operative also in weightbearing, pressure from clothes, shoes, or lying on a painful shoulder or hip.
3. Functional movement which encroaches on the painful range.

Headache triggers

In the upper cervical spine the trigger factors are more complex in their influence than those operative at other joints. Headache is triggered by a great diversity of factors, some of which are specific to certain individuals.

Positioning

As in any other joint, a position which stretches or compresses the painful structure of a subsymptomatic joint will render it symptomatic. Flexion of the lordotic spinal areas, for example the sitting position for the lumbar spine and head-on-neck flexion for the cervical spine which contains the headache-producing joints, is most often the unfavourable position. The flexed position is required in reading, study, desk work, needlework and other handicrafts. Many people who respond with headache to these circumstances think that the headache is caused by eyestrain but it is, in fact, caused by neck strain. Eyestrain as such does not produce a headache. The fixation of the head on the neck required for the sustained focusing of the eyes maintains the upper cervical spine in an unfavourable position, and it is this that precipitates the headache.

Even maintaining the head in a neutral position for any length of time may bring on a headache, e.g. driving or watching television. Sitting in an auditorium could involve some degree of neck extension. I recall a patient telling me that when she sat near the front of the church or cinema she got a headache but not if she sat near the back. This means that her neck was uncomfortable in some degree of extension but comfortable in a neutral or slightly flexed position. The opposite could be true for another person with a lesion, even if it involved the same level, where that joint could be uncomfortable in flexion and where extension could be the position of ease.

Headaches which come on overnight are probably due to an unfavourable position acquired during the night. Other headaches are relieved by the recumbent position and aggravated by the upright. It depends on the particular joint lesion. A position which is painful for one person could be the position of ease for another.

Pressure

A great many factors which involve pressure are potent triggers of headache. Localized oedema is not often one of them except in recent trauma when it is important to treat the oedema in order to reduce the pain.

When there is a painful lesion of the upper cervical articulations they become extraordinarily sensitive to pressure. Perhaps this is so because there is usually a certain amount of protective muscle spasm secondary to the lesion and when pressure from another source is added it causes the pain to spill over and the lesion becomes symptomatic. The merest finger pressure on such a joint can be unbelievably painful. The following passages from the works of other authors tie in with my own feeling that any situation which involves even the slightest pressure change near the headache lesion can precipitate the headache.

Maxwell (1966) writes: ‘Essentially, alterations of the intracranial hydrodynamics account for the majority of headaches’. I would like to insert ‘and suboccipital’ after ‘intracranial’. Suppose the disorder existing at the O/Cl joint is an irritable one, then any change in the hydrodynamics of its environment could become a potential headache trigger. This change in hydrodynamics could be brought about by cervical muscle contraction such as is experienced in stressful situations. Also premenstrually, fluid is retained in all the tissues throughout the body and thus also in the environment of the craniovertebral joints constituting a pressure increase.

Grieve (1981) writes: ‘The neck has been described as a triumph of packaging. There is little room for physical trespass by one tissue upon the territory of another’.

The following factors which commonly trigger headache must be considered in context with the foregoing. It is possible that the common denominator embodies the pressure factor.

Nervous tension

In stressful situations an adrenaline release causes, among other reactions, the cervical muscles to contract. If there is a pre-existing lesion in the cervical spine which could refer its pain as headache there will already be a protecting muscle spasm. The stress-induced muscle contraction is then added to this, thus multiplying the pressure which mechanically compresses the articular lesion and renders it symptomatic. The treatment of choice is not to eliminate the stress response, which is normal, but to improve the joint function. Muscular compression of normal joints does not give rise to pain. Everyone who is subjected to stress does not suffer headache.

Premenstrual fluid retention, hormonal changes during puberty, menopause, pregnancy, the birth control pill and headache which abates in old age

Headache is frequently related to menstruation, most commonly coming on or becoming worse premenstrually. I think that the effect of premenstrual fluid retention is operative throughout the body and so also exerts pressure in the closely packaged cervical region. Whatever the explanation, it is a fact that when a cervical headache has been successfully treated by means of mobilization, the patient will no longer experience premenstrual headache. We are, perhaps, more familiar with this situation when treating a lumbar lesion where the same principle applies. At puberty, the menopause and in pregnancy there are hormonally-induced tissue fluid fluctuations and in old age tissue fluid pressures fall.

Sinusitis and crying

Marmion (1957) wrote:

> ' . . . sinusitis is greatly overrated as a cause of headache. Examination and therapeutic procedures for the sinuses are commonly carried out in chronic headaches and seldom afford benefit. If there is an improvement in the headaches after such procedures, the reason is possibly that the congestion which was triggering the cervical headache is relieved'.

There is a difference between the pure sinusitis headache and the cervical headache which is triggered by congested nasal sinuses. In the absence of a cervical lesion, a sinus headache is localized to the area overlying the frontal and maxillary sinuses. It is not a severe pain but rather a feeling of discomfort and pressure.

It is not uncommon for a headache of primary cervical articular origin to be triggered or aggravated when the nasal sinuses are congested. The same headache can also be triggered by crying. The headache so triggered can be relieved by mobilizing the culpable vertebral joints. But what is hard to understand is that, when these joints are mobilized, the sinuses immediately drain. This is most noticeable when transverse pressure is applied to the tip of the transverse process of the atlas (*see* Chapter 10). As the patient sits up after the application of this technique her sinuses will start to drain.

Smoking, alcohol and other ingestants

The effect of smoking and drinking on headache invites speculation. Either can increase or trigger a headache in a headache susceptible person although one is a vasoconstrictor and the other a vasodilator. Perhaps Maxwell (1966) is approaching an explanation when he writes: 'Essentially alterations of the intracranial hydrodynamics account for the majority of headaches'. It seems probable that changes in intracranial hydrodynamics would also be effective at the craniovertebral joint and that factors which dilate and constrict blood vessels could set off an irritable lesion there. A decrease in pressure around this joint could be as irritating as an increase.

The headache triggered by alcohol could, of course, be a vascular headache where the pain arises from the vasodilation of the cranial vessels caused by the alcohol, but where such a headache is relieved by means of mobilizing the neck it seems that the alcohol must have triggered a cervical headache.

Blood pressure

It is debatable whether high blood pressure causes headache (*see* Chapter 2), but since many people seem to associate the two it is not impossible that the anxiety which is incumbent on hypertension could be responsible for sustained muscle contraction which activates a dormant cervical lesion. If this is the case then mobilization of the neck would relieve the headache.

Post lumbar puncture headache

The headache which often follows lumbar puncture is ascribed to the drop in cerebrospinal fluid pressure due to leakage. This is always stated to be the cause but the pain-producing mechanism is not spelled out. Graham (1964) writes that 'the headache that follows lumbar puncture has vascular components' and that they are related to the decreased volume of cerebrospinal fluid. Other components are suggested, for example that, rarely, there may be a meningeal reaction. It is also said that the patient is more likely to develop headache if it is 'suggested' to him in advance. Also that:

> '... tense patients may have a post-puncture headache of the muscle contraction or vascular variety such as may follow a period of anxiety related to any needling procedure. If they develop this type of headache and have also lost fluid via the puncture hole, the combination may act synergistically to produce a severe headache, present even in the horizontal position and accentuated by standing up – a ''combined'' post lumbar puncture headache syndrome' (Graham, 1964).

As there does not seem to be one definitive pathogenic mechanism for post lumbar puncture headache I would like to add to the possibilities. I think that any one of the aforementioned components could set off a craniovertebral joint lesion as a contributing cause for headache. In fact, I think that this is the underlying mechanism of the muscle contraction headache mentioned by Graham (1964).

Interestingly, not all post lumbar puncture subjects develop a headache. Perhaps they have no cervical lesion.

Personalized triggers

There seems to be a group of triggers which does not fit into any of the foregoing headings. They are highly personalized in their actions and only trigger headaches in certain individuals.

One example is ingestants. Although dairy products, chocolate and red wine are the common ingestant triggers of those who are sensitive to ingestants at all, some headaches are set off by white wine and not red, others by beer and not by wine and yet others by alcohol in any form. Some people respond in this way to, say, fried food and one patient I recall always had a headache after eating food that had been frozen and reheated.

Researchers have studied the chemical effects of substances contained in the common headache-producing ingestants on the vasoreaction which takes place in migraine subjects, but with inconclusive results. To the best of my knowledge no research has been done on ingestants as a trigger of cervical headache. It seems that certain people have specific intolerance to particular ingestants and that these provoke a systemic reaction and a feeling often described by the layman as 'biliousness'. In those of them that have a primary headache-producing lesion, whether articular or vascular, this feeling is followed by headache. People call it a 'sick headache'.

Other personalized triggers include lights, either bright, moving, flickering, flashing, fluorescent or coloured; loud noise and certain odours are not uncommon; and there was more than one who reported that asbestos heaters in a room could start a headache.

We recently had a patient, a young man who had suffered a skull fracture about a year previously, and since had been plagued with headache which unfailingly came on when the sky was overcast and went away when it was clear. After mobilization of the painful cervical joints (which were damaged by the blow which fractured his skull) the headache abated altogether and no longer came on when there were clouds in the sky.

I think that anything that the headache-prone person finds personally irritating, whether it is a physiological intolerance to particular ingestants or inhalants, or a psychological aversion, seems to result in headache. Perhaps it is that a factor which irritates sets up a sustained cervical muscle contraction in response to the discomfort or irritation being suffered and so triggers the painful joints.

This chapter does not represent established medical opinion, but rather the author's attempt to understand clinical evidence. These factors are reported by patients as being triggers of their headache, and when the headache has been abated by means of manipulating the cervical spine, these same triggers which remain present in their lives no longer result in headache.

This thinking could be applied to factors often reported as being potent triggers of headache, e.g. inflammatory conditions, intracranial disorders, changes of altitude, headstands, dehydration and hangover headache. I think that none of these factors constitutes a prime cause of headache but that they set off symptoms from the primary headache-causing lesion whether this is vascular or arthrotic or both.

In cases where this lesion is minimal, these factors if intense or protracted may give rise to a mild headache. People with such minimal lesions commonly report 'occasional' headache (less often than one per month) and describe them as 'not severe' and say that a simple analgesic gives sure relief (TPP = 3/15) (Edeling, 1980).

The more advanced the pathology at the culpable joints the more easily the symptoms are evoked (because they become increasingly pressure-sensitive) and therefore the pain occurs more frequently. Correspondingly the ensuing pain is more severe and requires more and more complex analgesics until a stage is reached when the pain is continuous, frequently severe and unresponsive to analgesics (TPP = 15/15). At this fully developed stage the pain can be totally relieved by the treatment to be taught in this book. The interesting thing is that as the syndrome abates the trigger factors become less potent or quite impotent as headache triggers, as they were before the onset of the syndrome in the same individual or in other individuals who do not have a subsymptomatic cervical condition. These subjects are then able to resume their normal lifestyle without the need to manipulate their environment in order to avoid headache triggers.

References

Edeling, J. (1980) The subjective assessment of pain in orthopaedic joint problems. *South African Journal of Physiotherapy*, **36**, 13–17

Graham, J. R. (1964) Treatment of non-migrainous vascular headache. In Friedman, A. P., ed., *Modern Treatment* (Symposium on the Treatment of Headache), Vol. 1, No. 6, p. 1439. Harper and Row, New York

Grieve, G. P. (1981) *Common Vertebral Problems*. Churchill Livingstone, Edinburgh

Marmion, D. E. (1957) The physical basis of headache. *The Practitioner*, **178**, 455–465

Maxwell, H. (1966) Pathological physiology of headache. In *Migraine*, Chapter V. John Wright, Bristol

7

Subjective assessment of pain

In the examination of any physical disorder the practitioner tries to reconcile subjective information with objective findings. If the condition involves the locomotive parts, the therapist will try to define the problem in terms of joint or muscle dysfunction. Often the exact nature of the pathology has not been defined and then trial treatment will be directed at effecting an improvement in signs and symptoms (Maitland, 1986). More weight is usually afforded to the signs, or objective findings, because these are more readily measurable and therefore of more scientific value (Edeling, 1980).

In cases where the subjective and objective examination are not equally informative the therapist is obliged to depend largely, and at times totally, on the one or the other. In such cases it will be clear that more time must be given to extricating every possible bit of information from the sources available.

Therapists are often confronted with this situation in cases where the overriding complaint is that of pain, as is the case in cervical headaches. The underlying pathology may be of a degenerative nature such as osteoarthrosis and so we do not aim to arrest or cure it but direct our efforts to relieving the aspect of the pathology that bothers the patient most and that is usually pain.

In such conditions pain is usually accompanied by joint stiffness or limitation of physiological or accessory movement. When this is so, measurement of the restriction forms an important part of the objective examination and the measured improvement in movement is used to evaluate the effectiveness of the trial treatment (Maitland, 1986).

It is quite common to find in headache patients with severe pain that there is no measurable limitation of physiological movement. There is, in these cases, painful limitation of a particular accessory movement which could help identify the site of the lesion, but in joints where the possibility of accessory movement is of a minute range an estimate of the degree of restriction could not be made with a great degree of accuracy. It is, in my experience, not a very helpful parameter for purposes of reassessment.

If, therefore, therapists are to have any chance of therapeutically relieving the pain in such cases they must make full use of all the available information, especially the patient's subjective account of pain. Many practitioners do not consider a subjective report of pain to be of much scientific value because it is not considered to be measurable. But when it becomes the only available parameter, ways must be found to use it. It is my experience that when patients are questioned in a methodical manner, they bear valuable testimony about their pain. I have established a system with which I evaluate my own patients and record comparable parameters. It has proved to be dependable and helpful for purposes of assessment and reassessment and I recommend its use.

It is necessary to elicit and *record* a total pain pattern (TPP) at first interview which includes a retrospective pattern beginning, perhaps, many years before and leading up to the pattern present at the time of presentation. The TPP will be unique to each patient.

Guiding principles

1. The TPP often suggests the diagnosis (*see* Chapters 2 and 9).
2. The main purpose of recording a TPP is to have a standard for comparison after treatment. In this way it will be possible to detect early marginal changes and so be able to evaluate the effectiveness of trial treatment.
3. There is admittedly no reliable way of comparing the subjective intensity of one person's pain with that of another. A patient is, however, well able to compare the intensity of her own pain at different times. The patient's report of the varying intensities and absence of her own pain are recorded for subsequent comparison. Every other clinical feature that can be extracted is also recorded. Many of these clinical features can be used as additional or alternative reassessment points.
4. The TPP of the cervical headache, if adequately taken, will portray the increasing severity of the pain syndrome up to the time of presentation, the initial response to treatment and the steady decrease until discharge. It will also enable the therapist to judge to what extent the improvement is maintained at subsequent follow-up assessment.
5. If the record is incomplete, attempts at reassessment are likely to be confusing and misleading.

Total pain pattern (TPP)

Distribution

The patient should be asked to indicate, using a finger, the area of the worst pain, the extent and manner of radiation or spread and any other related or unrelated areas of pain; also where the pain usually begins or is first felt. The patient may say that under certain circumstances it is in one area and under others, elsewhere. These areas should be carefully drawn in on a chart with suitable annotations and, before going further, the patient should be shown the chart and requested to confirm the pain distribution recorded and to check notes for accuracy (*see Figure 7.1*). Changes in the pain distribution pattern could mean that treatment is having an effect on the pain.

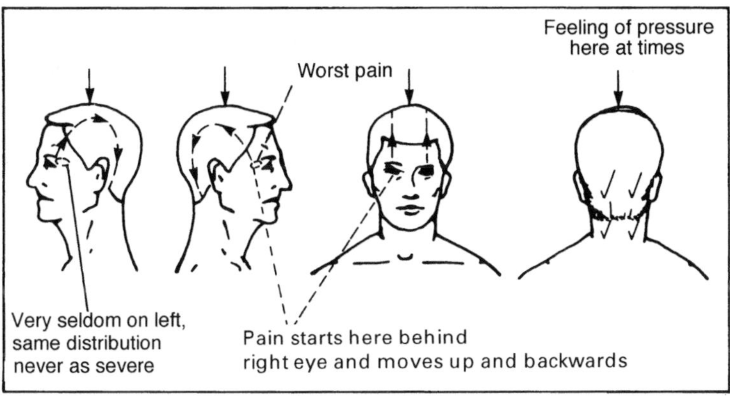

Figure 7.1 One example of a pain chart

Nature of pain

A clear distinction must be made between the nature (or quality) of pain and the intensity of pain. If the question is put as follows: 'What does the pain feel like?', the patient will often tell how severe it is. It is better to ask: 'What does the pain feel like?', and add: 'I don't mean how bad is it but what sort of pain is it?'. If a spontaneous reply is not forthcoming, she should be helped by saying: 'Does it throb, or is there a feeling of pressure or burning about it?' and she will then understand and respond by saying: 'Oh no, it never throbs or burns – it's just a gnawing pain' or whatever the case may be. Some patients do not know that there are various qualities to pain. They think that what they feel is pain and that all pain feels as theirs does.

Periodicity (P)

When there is an established periodicity pattern to the occurrence of the pain of headache, this forms the most useful feature for measuring improvement during the course of treatment. Mostly it is a very simple matter. If a patient has had a continuous pain for a long period and during the course of treatment the pain becomes intermittent and finally abates, one need not perform mental gymnastics in order to assess improvement.

All too often there are, however, confusing factors that bedevil assessment. This may cause one to abandon the only effective treatment because one had not been aware of the initial marginal improvement in the periodicity pattern.

It is useful to grade the periodicity pattern from P = 1/5 to P = 5/5.

Grade P 1/5 = Pain on one day per month or less
P 2/5 = Pain on two or more days per month
P 3/5 = Pain on one or more days a week
P 4/5 = Daily but intermittent pain
P 5/5 = Continuous pain.

Reassessment

If a P 5/5 pain abates altogether for even a very short time after treatment it is no longer a P 5/5 but a P 4/5. If a P 4/5 pain skips a day, it becomes a P 3/5, etc. When pain periodicity patterns do not readily conform to this system because they are erratic, one is still able to use it but it requires much more skill on the part of the assessor.

Intensity (I)

The subjective intensity of pain can also be graded from I 1/5 to I 5/5.

Grade I 1/5 = Mild pain
I 2/5 = More than mild pain but tolerable
I 3/5 = Moderately severe pain
I 4/5 = Severe pain
I 5/5 = Intolerable, perhaps suicidal pain.

Patients are often quick to match their pain intensity to one of the above grades. If they are not they should be asked what they feel like and how it affects them when the pain is at its *worst*. This usually unleashes a vivid description of the impact of the pain on the individual. The therapist must then interpret this impact:

I 1/5: Is it a barely perceptible pain: of nuisance value only?
I 3/5: Is it a strong pain? Is the pain affecting the patient's daily life? Does it disrupt her lifestyle, work, domestic or social life?
I 5/5: Is it incapacitating? Is the pain completely intolerable and destructive? Is life totally engulfed in unrelieved severe pain? Are there hints of despair, suicide? Could you, the therapist, live with such pain?

Assess accordingly. Do you consider this pain to be a Grade I 1/5, I 3/5 or I 5/5, or does it fall in between, i.e. I 2/5 or I 4/5? This becomes the therapist's 'measure' of the intensity of pain.

Although the pain fluctuates in intensity, how often is it maximal?

Response to analgesics (R) – self-administered or prescribed

It seems that the response of pain to analgesia often depends on the stage of the pathology which is responsible for the pain. If one considers the kind of pain which arises from painful joint restriction, as in cervical vertebral headaches, it will be found that as the joint condition deteriorates analgesics become progressively less effective. Later if the physiotherapy treatment is improving the condition of the joint, analgesics become more and more effective. As this fact emerged repeatedly in patient's reports I decided to include response to analgesics as yet another parameter for 'measuring' the improvement of the headache condition. Very often assessment of the response to analgesics is helpful when reassessment of other factors is inconclusive.

For example, if initially a patient reports that no amount of analgesics totally relieves her pain but two paracetamol will lessen it for an hour or so and after a couple of trial treatments she tells you that her pain went away completely for several hours with the same dose, this indicates an improvement. Response to analgesics may also be graded R 1/5 to R 5/5;

Grade R l/5 = Pain abates readily with small dose of simple analgesic
R 2/5 = Pain is lessened but does not go away with simple analgesic
R 3/5 = Pain is totally relieved by compound analgesic
R 4/5 = Pain is lessened but does not go away with a large dose of compound analgesic
R 5/5 = No dose of any analgesic has any effect at all on the pain.

Precipitating and aggravating factors

In this instance the therapist wishes to know from the patient what it is that brings on the pain or what makes it worse when it is already there. When there is a spontaneous reply it should be recorded verbatim and earmarked for later comparison. If one or more of these factors become impotent after treatment, this signifies improvement in or cure of the pain-producing condition.

It will be found that the patient with a long established pattern of pain will readily supply these factors. Those with patterns of more recent onset will be less able to do so. If a patient says she doesn't know what brings on her pain, one should gently probe and give examples of the factors that many other patients have reported in answer to these questions. This will help her to understand what is being sought and she may be able to supply the relevant information, perhaps not immediately but perhaps at the next visit when she has had a chance to register the precipitants. Sometimes, however, there is no discernible trigger factor.

Associated or concomitant symptoms

The patient should be asked: 'Apart from the pain, do you have other sensations that seem to come and go with the pain, or when the pain is very bad?'. These must be recorded verbatim. If she says that she hears a sound in her left ear like a cricket chirruping, or like bubbles, these should not be transcribed and recorded as 'tinnitus'. Record the patient's words. Associated symptoms are less useful as a yardstick for measuring improvement as they have no numerical potential, but the TTP is incomplete if you do not know about them. It is here that warnings of pathology which lie beyond the scope of physiotherapy may be picked up. These replies should be adequately recorded because these symptoms will sometimes abate before the pain does in which case they indicate improvement.

History

To complete the TPP, a retrospective history should be taken which should cover aspects such as the following:

1. Initial onset of this pain pattern.
2. Progression over years/months/days.
3. Aetiology – whether trauma, disease, strain, stress, surgery, pregnancy, occupational posture, etc., can be related to the pre-syndrome stage.
4. Previous medical examinations (relating specifically to the headache), diagnoses, treatment and response to such treatments; lay practitioners consulted and result of their treatment; previous physiotherapy and modalities employed, with result.
5. Familial factors, childhood allergies and motion sickness.

Questioning technique

1. Allow plenty of time for the first interview, about 45 minutes. (With experience this time will become less, but it should never be deliberately hurried.)
2. Use recording sheets with standard headings in order to achieve an ordered line of questioning but do not be rigid if the patient offers information that does not seem to fit the form. Record it under a heading called 'miscellaneous' or 'points of interest'. An example of a recording sheet is shown in the Appendix (p. 162).
3. Do not restrict the patient to brief answers. Encourage her, at some stage, to just 'tell me about your pain'. This elicits a useful impression of just how much the pain intrudes on her life. If she rambles on too much she should be guided back to answering more direct questions.
4. Often patients are embarrassed about describing bizarre symptoms. They are afraid that the interviewer will think that they are imagining things or exaggerating. The therapist should seem interested but unalarmed when they tell of strange sensations which frighten them. They should be reassured where necessary.
5. The therapist should not seem to be critical when questioning about analgesics or other drugs. The patient will think that the therapist is going to restrict her drug taking and will give evasive answers. She is already worried about side-effects but cannot face the pain without analgesics. She must be given to understand that all that is required is information for later comparison. If, later, she needs fewer pain killers, her pain-producing condition is improving. Also, if the same analgesic which previously gave no or little relief later gives some or total relief, the condition is improving.
6. When asking about aggravating or precipitating factors and/or associated symptoms the therapist must be matter-of-fact in his manner. Patients with a chronic headache, for instance, frequently have concomitant symptoms that terrify them, e.g. strange noises in their ears, a feeling of constriction in the throat, dysphasia and visual disturbances. These symptoms should be asked for in an ordinary way, recorded and the patient should be reassured if she seems anxious about them. If the patient says: 'You probably won't believe me but my pain is worst when my mother-in-law visits', believe her and record this fact. If later, in the course of treatment she reports a visit from mother-in-law with no ensuing headache, the therapist may assume that it is the condition that has improved and not the mother-in-law. If you are

alerted by a report, do not alarm the patient but make a note to check the following:

(a) Is this a familiar report in your clinical situation? Is it perhaps indicative of some condition which does not lie within the scope of the therapist?

(b) Has the patient told her doctor about it? Whether or not, it might be wise for the therapist to discuss it with the doctor before proceeding with further treatment.

(c) Has the patient been seen by an appropriate specialist and have the necessary diagnostic tests been carried out? If so, there is seldom cause for alarm.

7. It is often helpful to record, verbatim, descriptive words or phrases used by the patient. These should not be transcribed. When reassessing at a later date use the same word or phrase which was recorded at the first visit. This enables the patient to identify the sensation which she originally described. She will at once be able to compare her present sensations or pain reliably and to say, quite definitely, for example: 'I no longer have that dreadful scalding pain, it's just a dull ache now', etc.
8. If the patient finds a question difficult to answer, do not press her. Help her by:

   (a) Rephrasing the question.

   (b) Telling her what you, as a therapist, are seeking to establish.

   (c) Saying the answer need not be exact but approximate, e.g. she can remember having a headache for the first time 'about fifteen years ago' is adequate for your purposes.

   (d) Passing on to the next question, saying that it is not important.
9. If the patient, at the first visit, is in severe pain do not subject her to prolonged questioning. Try to give some relief with soothing modalities of treatment and leave the TPP till the severe attack has passed.
10. When questioning for response to treatment never seem to be disappointed or sceptical when a patient reports a negative response. She should be questioned further to ensure that there had been no marginal improvement which she might have thought to be irrelevant. If there was none, do not discredit the patient's report but try alternative treatment techniques until there is a positive response. The patient must understand that the therapist is seeking the truth and not gratification.

Assessment based on TPP

When attempting to arrive at a numerical estimate of a pain syndrome one must consider more than one parameter. Periodicity (P), intensity (I) and response to analgesics (R) are used according to the grading shown under the relevant headings.

Pain should be sought of in terms of 'quantity of pain' (*see Figures 12.1–12.3*), i.e. how much pain is there for what proportion of the day, week, month, year? The quantity of pain is the sum of P and I and the indices for each of these are added together. It is not sufficient to estimate the severity of the syndrome in terms of pain intensity alone. If one adds the R index the numerical index gains another dimension. The TPP is the sum of the three indices and an increase or decrease in any one of them will be reflected in a numerical reduction of the TPP.

Example

A typical but uncomplicated pattern is depicted as follows:

A woman aged 53 complains of daily headache. She wakes without it but it comes on mid-morning and builds up. By midday it is so severe that she is unable to concentrate on her work as a typist. She is obliged to take two compound analgesics but these do not totally relieve her pain but reduce it to a level which allows her to continue her work through the afternoon.

Estimate of the TPP at this stage:
P = 4/5, I = 3/5, R = 4/5, TPP = 11/15

She says that she has suffered headaches for very many years, possibly since puberty, but that they had only been as bad as they are now for the past four years. During her high school years she remembers having headaches at examination times but they were mild compared with her present headaches and were totally relieved by an aspirin tablet.

Estimate of the TPP at that stage:
P = 1/5, I = 1/5, R = 1/5; TPP = 3/15

After the birth of her second child (at age 23) the headaches became worse. She remembers that she often had headaches when the children were small and that they were no longer mild. Aspirin had less and less effect.

Estimate of TPP over these intervening years:
P = 2–3/5, I = 2/5, R = 2–3/5; TPP = 6–8/15

Four years ago, after a minor whiplash injury, the headaches worsened to the present level which has been established as:
P = 4/5, I = 3/5, R = 4/5; TPP = 11/15

After a few initial treatments she reports that her headache came on as usual but went away for several hours after taking her usual tablets.

Now:
P = 4/5, I = 3/5, R = 3/5; TPP = 10/15

The therapist continued with the same treatment techniques, increasing the dosage as the symptoms lessened. The patient then reported that her headache skipped a day, but when it came on the following day it was of the same intensity, but was again totally relieved by the same tablets.

Now:
P = 3/5, I = 3/5, R = 3/5; TPP = 9/15

Subsequent reports reveal diminishing P, I and R indices.

When the patient has had no headache for a month:
P = ?0 or 1/5, I = 0, R = 0; TPP = ?0 or 1/15

This pattern may be graphically depicted as shown in *Figure 7.2*.

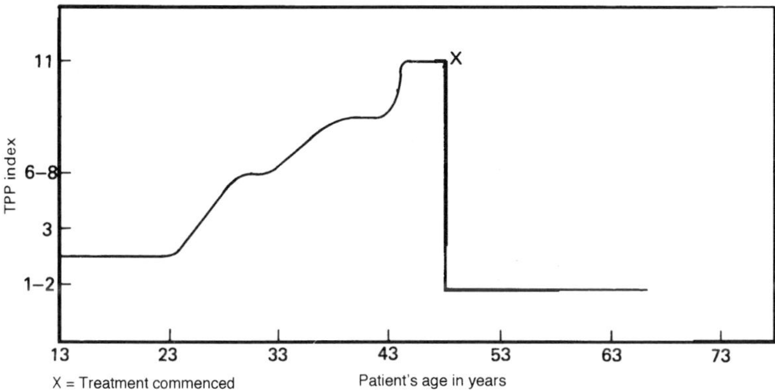

Figure 7.2 Pain diagram

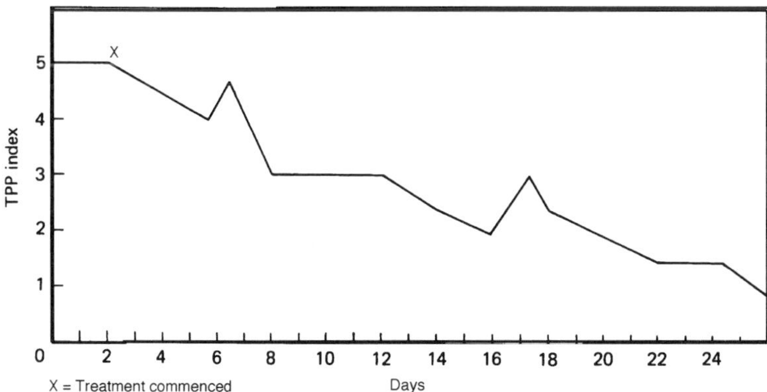

Figure 7.3 Pain diagram

It is of critical importance to be able to judge the initial marginal response to trial treatment techniques. If this is not correctly perceived or correctly interpreted, the particular technique which had produced this marginal response might be discarded instead of pursued. Furthermore, after the initial favourable response to treatment, there is usually an overall decline in the TPP (and therefore of the syndrome) but it might not always be a linear decline. The improvement could be interspersed with peaks of seeming recurrences. If the therapist has an accurate record it will be clear to him and to the patient that these are peaks in a rapidly declining linear relationship (*see Figure 7.3*).

References

Edeling, J. (1980) The subjective assessment of pain in orthopaedic joint problems. *South African Journal of Physiotherapy*, **36**, 13–17

Maitland, G. D. (1986) *Vertebral Manipulation*, 5th edn., p. vii. Butterworths, London

8

Physical examination

In painful joint conditions the examiner would expect to find limitation of physiological movement which involves the culpable joint. For example, when a lumbar paravertebral joint is responsible for severe pain radiating down the leg, lumbar movement, often lumbar flexion, would be found to be grossly limited. So certainly would he expect to find this, that if the lumbar movements were found to be of a normal range in such a case, he would exclude the lumbar spine as a possible source and seek the pain elsewhere. The same would apply to a case of brachialgia. Certain cervical movement, usually rotation or side flexion, will be found to be blocked.

In examining the cervical spine for a possible source of severe headache, this expected limitation of physiological movement is not always apparent. Frequently, even in the presence of severe headache emanating from the cervical spine, the physiological cervical movements appear to be of normal range. This might be explained by the fact that there is a large discrepancy of possible movement in the three directions (flexion/extension, lateral flexion and axial rotation) at the O/C1 and C1/C2 joints.

Whereas Hohl (1964) states that 'the atlanto-occipital joint permits only flexion and extension but the more complex atlanto-axial joint allows flexion and extension, rotation, vertical approximation and lateral gliding.', White and Panjabi (1978) show:

At O/C1	Flexion/extension	– 13° (moderate)
	Lateral flexion	– 8° (moderate)
	Axial rotation	– 0° (negligible)
At C1/C2	Flexion/extension	– 10° (moderate)
	Lateral flexion	– 0° (negligible)
	Axial rotation	– 47° (extensive)

The almost imperceptible movement of axial rotation at O/C1 and of lateral flexion at C1/C2, however, does not rule out the presence of accessory movement at these levels. Accessory movement in any joint is of very small amplitude. If this small movement potential is further diminished by disease process there remains no movement at all. When physiological movement tests are performed the joint responsible for the pain will not move and its pain will only be detected if its passive accessory movement is tested. Failure to examine accessory movement could mislead the examiner into excluding the cervical spine as a source of the headache.

The therapist will find that in cases where the head pain seems to be unrelated to the neck, active movement of the neck will not be restricted or painful. The lesion will then most likely be found, by means of palpating the passive intervertebral movement, to be at the atlanto-occipital joint.

When the pain in the head stems from the suboccipital area and radiates up the occiput and over the vertex to the prefrontal area, the lesion is likely to be found at the atlanto-axial joint. In this case active rotation to the left or the right might be limited, but possibly only when overpressure is passively applied after the end of the voluntary range.

When there is neck pain as well as headache, both the upper cervical spine (O/C1/C2) and also the mid and/or lower cervical spine are implicated and all of these articulations will need to be examined and treated to clear signs in order to rid the patient of headache and neck pain.

In cases of isolated head pain where there is no complaint of suboccipital or neck pain, little will be gained from the testing of cervical physiological movement. Palpation and passive intervertebral movement testing will provide the positive signs which will indicate the joint to be treated and the technique which is likely to be effective. Physiological movements should, however, be tested for completeness of the examination.

By the time a comprehensive subjective examination has been recorded one would know whether it will be necessary to concentrate more on movement or palpation testing.

Physical testing

This follows on the assessment and planning stage suggested in the previous chapter.

Always:

1. Observe and record how the patient looks and feels at that moment before objective examining procedures are begun, for example:
   - face looks pale and drawn; ptosis left eye/eyes dull
   - shoulders slightly hunched, poking chin
   - c/o pain over left eye, as chart, moderate intensity
   - feeling of nausea/dizziness (slight).
2. Test the patency of the vertebral artery with the patient sitting:
   (a) Sustained maximum available rotation to the left and then to the right, asking about a feeling of dizziness after each movement and observing for nystagmus.
   (b) Sustained extension – assess as before.
   (c) Sustained extension combined with side flexion to the left and then to the right – assess as before.
   Repeat these three procedures with the patient lying supine. Record and asterisk positive findings. Positive signs of vertebral artery insufficiency found and recorded here would influence the therapist's decision to manipulate (Grade V) at any future stage of treatment.
3. With the patient in a comfortable sitting position, decide on the basis of the foregoing subjective examination and assessment which of the following procedures to follow or omit.

Physiological movement test (Maitland, 1986)

General cervical flexion (*Figure 8.1a*).
General cervical flexion with overpressure (*Figure 8.1b*).
General cervical extension (*Figure 8.2a*).
General cervical extension with overpressure (*Figure 8.2b*).

When general flexion or extension produces pain it may be desirable to discover whether the pain stems from the upper or lower cervical spine. This differentiation may be achieved by testing as follows:

Lower cervical flexion combined with upper cervical extension. In this movement the chin is stretched out forward (*Figure 8.3*).
Upper cervical flexion combined with lower cervical extension, in which the chin is pulled in and back (*Figure 8.4*).
Left and right flexion.
Left and right rotation.

Each of these movements should be tested with the application of overpressure if no pain is elicited through range.

If no pain was elicited during the performance of any of the foregoing movement tests, test the following combined movements.

Upper cervical quadrant to the left

According to Maitland (1986):

> 'The physiotherapist stands at the patient's left side and guides her head into extension, applying pressure to localize the movement to the upper cervical joints. This is done by grasping the patient's chin from underneath in the left hand and her forehead in the right. At the same time her trunk should be stabilized by the physiotherapist's arm from behind and his side from in front while applying pressure through his hands to flex the lower cervical spine with the head held in extension. While head extension is maintained, rotation to the left is added. The axis of rotation has changed from the vertical when the head is held in the upright position to almost horizontal when the head is in full extension. It is the head which is turned and the technique is to produce oscillatory movements so that the limit of the rotatory range can be felt. When the head is fully turned towards the physiotherapist he then adds the lateral flexion component. The lateral flexion movement involves tilting the crown of the patient's head towards him and her chin away from him. This movement is also performed in an oscillatory fashion until the limit of range is reached. This is a difficult test movement to carry out and much practice is necessary to perform it well.'

Full and pain-free performance of the foregoing tests do not exclude the cervical articulations as the source of headache. Further tests may be positive.

The examination of the cervical spine is described by Maitland (1986). I have reproduced from his text that which is relevant for this chapter, and added or modified certain sections which relate specifically or exclusively to the symptom of headache.

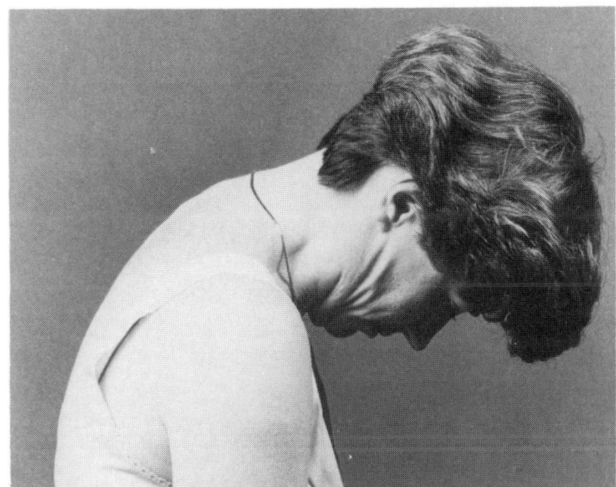

Figure 8.1 (a) General cervical flexion

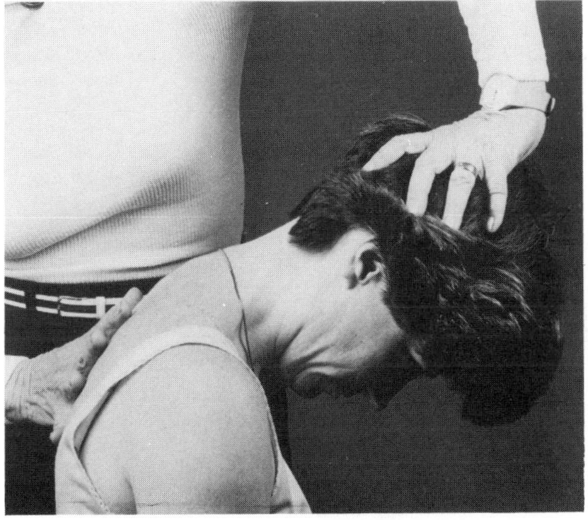

Figure 8.1 (b) The same movement with overpressure

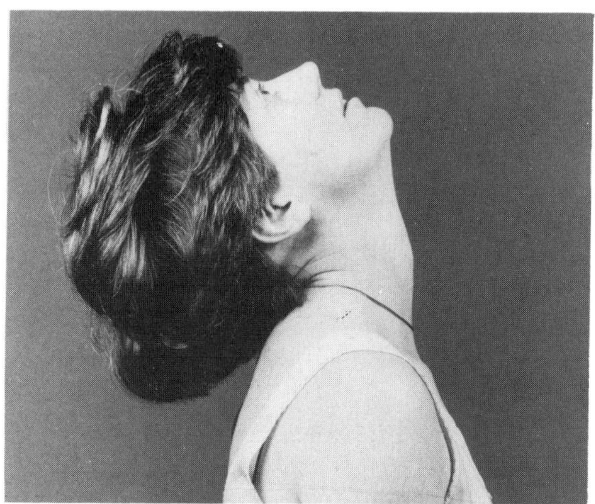

Figure 8.2 (a) General cervical extension

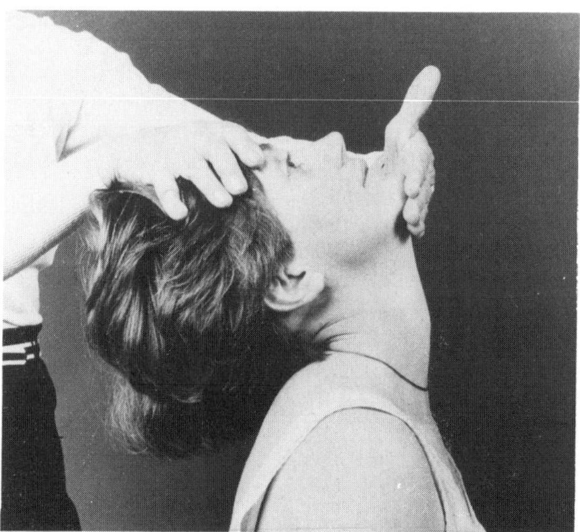

Figure 8.2 (b) The same movement with overpressure

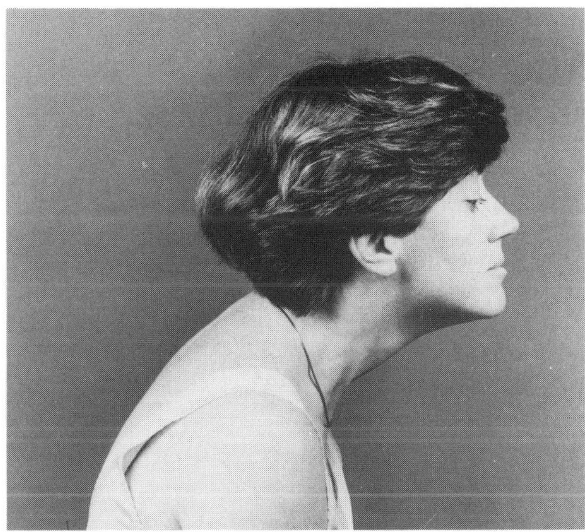

Figure 8.3 (a) Lower cervical flexion combined with upper cervical extension

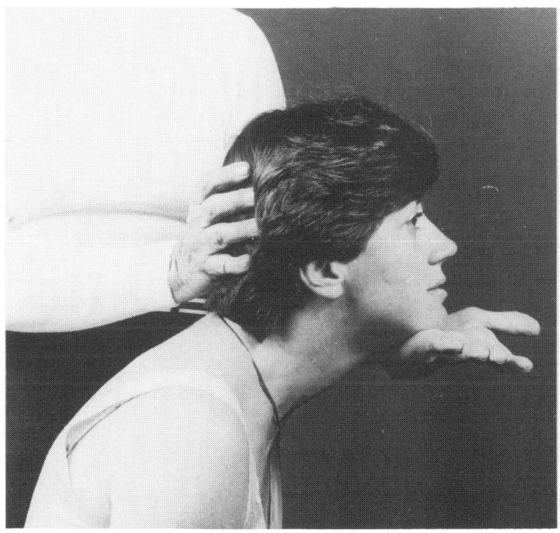

Figure 8.3 (b) The same movement with overpressure

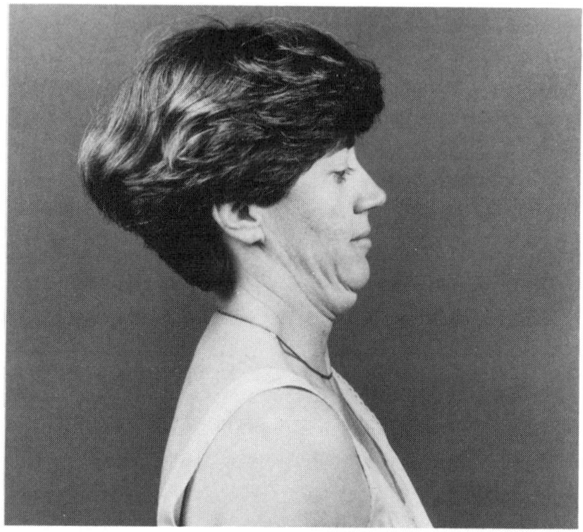

Figure 8.4 (a) Upper cervical flexion combined with lower cervical extension

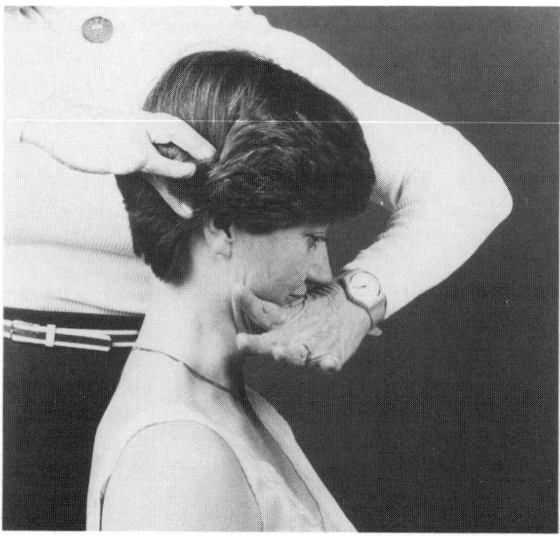

Figure 8.4 (b) The same movement with overpressure

Intervertebral tests by palpation

'In relation to examining the normality or otherwise of intervertebral movements, the most important techniques are those which follow. It is possible for a patient's physiological movements to appear normal yet the palpation tests for intervertebral movement will reveal positive appropriate joint signs.

Under the above heading the examination includes the following tests:

1. Skin temperature and sweating
2. Soft tissue tension
3. Position of vertebrae
4. Movement of vertebrae.

The four procedures given above constitute the usual routine palpation for vertebral conditions. This routine should be followed but with the following modifications when examining for cervical headache. Palpation at the first visit must be kept to a minimum. If the headache is coming from the occipito-atlanto-axial articulations (O/C1/C2) they will be extraordinarily sensitive to the touch and palpatory pressure is likely to cause a subsequent exacerbation of pain, however carefully carried out. For this reason it is best to palpate for pain only, omitting, at this stage, palpation for position of the vertebrae and even for restriction of range of movement. The source of the headache will be extremely painful to a Grade 1 pressure. It is unnecessary to increase the grade in order to find it. The point of pressure at which the pain response is greatest is likely to be the source of the headache and should be treated as suggested in Chapter 11.

When the spine is being examined the patient lies prone and the skin is checked for sweating and temperature. Palpation for muscle spasm and general tissue tension then follows. Finally, before testing intervertebral movement, the position of the vertebrae should be assessed in relation to adjacent vertebrae. Not too much importance should be placed on abnormalities found on this assessment as they are only relevant if they can be verified by radiography. As there are some differences in procedure for testing some levels of the spine, each will be described separately. Description of the tests for movement will then follow.'

Position tests

'**C1.** The patient lies prone and rests her forehead on her hands while the physiotherapist palpates between the spinous processes of C2 and the occiput to ascertain whether the posterior tubercle of C1 is palpable. From this point he palpates bilaterally through the relaxed suboccipital muscles, moving laterally until the tip of the transverse process is reached. The relationship which each side of C1 bears to the occiput and to C2 should be assessed. This finding is assisted by also palpating the tip of C1 laterally to assess its relationship to the anterior border of the mastoid process.'

'**C2–C7.** The spinous processes are unreliable as the sole source of information regarding position of the vertebrae. They frequently veer to one side without there being any deviation of the body of the vertebrae, and absence of one or other terminal tubercle is common. However, as they are accessible they are palpated first. If a spinous process is not central, the articular pillar and interlaminar space are then palpated to see if their position indicates any rotation or lateral flexion. The articular pillar is also palpated laterally, and the transverse processes anterolaterally. Apophyseal joint exostoses can be clearly felt. With practice it is possible to appreciate even a small loss of normal cervical lordosis.'

Movement tests

'Testing movement by palpation involves techniques which are used for treatment as well as examination. The test seeks information not only of range but also of the 'end-feel' of the range, and the quality of any resistance or muscle spasm which may be present. Such information is determined for both the physiological movements and the accessory movements of gapping, rocking, and shearing or gliding.

The passive intervertebral movements are produced by pressure against palpable parts of the vertebrae and these pressures should be applied at the right speed to appreciate the movement of the vertebrae in relation to adjacent vertebrae. If the pressure is applied as a single slow pressure, the vertebral movement will not be appreciated at all; if it is applied too quickly it can only be interpreted as shaking. However, if the pressure is applied then relaxed and reapplied and repeated two or three times a second, the amount of movement which can take place will be readily appreciated.

When examining movement the first pressures should be applied extremely gently. When a section of the spine is being treated in this way no more than two or three gentle pressures are applied to each vertebra in turn. If there is no pain response to the gentle movements the amplitude and depth of the movement is increased, still only two or three pressures per vertebra. The testing should be repeated more deeply until pain or abnormality is detected or until the movement achieved indicates that the joint has painless range in this direction. If pain is produced during movement, or if physical resistance or protective muscle contraction are encountered during the movement, their extent should be assessed. Occasionally a full assessment may not be possible until the second examination because pain with movement may not be evident until the joint has reacted to the first examination.

The three primary directions in which the pressures are applied are as follows:

1. Postero-anteriorly on the spinous process (*Figure 8.5a*).
2. Postero-anteriorly on the articular pillar (*Figure 8.5b*).
3. Transversely on the lateral surface of the spinous process (Figure 8.5c).

The test can then be further defined to determine the joint disturbance in greater detail by varying the direction of the above three pressures.

Postero-anteriorly on the spinous process, the direction of the pressures can be varied between an inclination towards the patient's:

1. head (*Figure 8.6a*)
2. feet (*Figure 8.6b*).

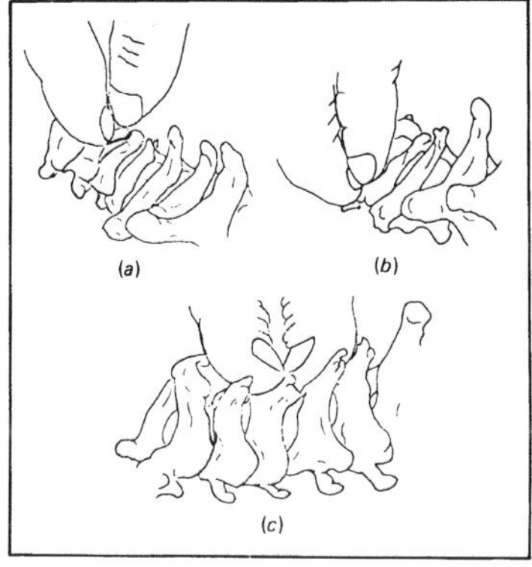

Figure 8.5 (a) Postero-anterior pressure on the spinous process; (b) postero-anterior pressure on the articular pillar; (c) transverse pressure on the lateral surface of the spinous process

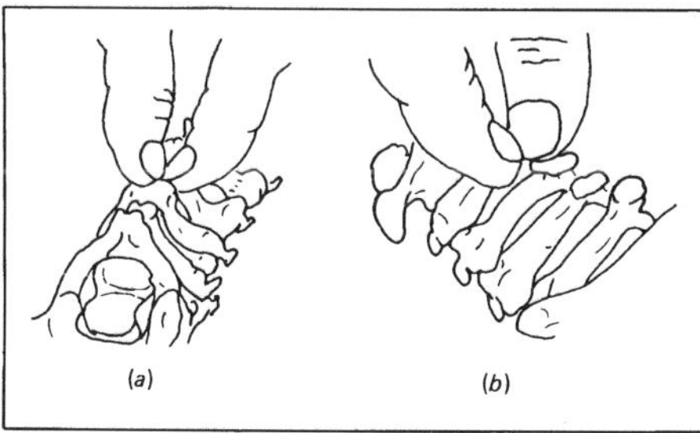

Figure 8.6 Postero-anterior pressure on the spinous process (a) inclined towards the patient's head; (b) inclined towards the patient's feet

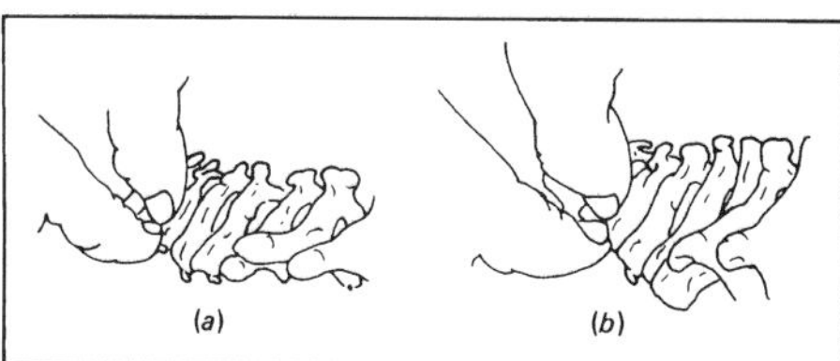

Figure 8.7 Postero-anterior pressure on the articular pillar (a) inclined laterally away from the spinous process; (b) inclined medially towards the spinous process

Postero-anteriorly over the articular pillar, this can be varied in the two directions suggested above and also:

3. laterally away from the spinous process (*Figure 8.7a*)
4. medially towards the spinous process (*Figure 8.7b*).

Transverse pressures against the spinous process can be applied as in 1 and 2 above and also:

5. It is even more important to vary the pressure from being applied transversely against the lateral surface of the spinous process, through an arc which ends as a postero-anterior pressure against the lamina or articular pillar of the same side of the vertebra (*Figure 8.8*).

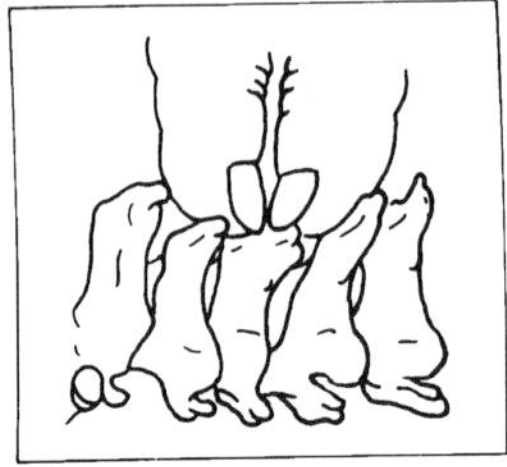

Figure 8.8 Transverse pressure against the spinous process inclined postero-anteriorly

As well as varying the angles of pressure applied to the vertebra, the point of contact should be varied by pressure on C2, then on C3 and then lastly on C2/3 joint line.

These tests carried out effectively will reveal not only the intervertebral joint at fault and the movement of the joint which is affected but also the manner in which each movement is affected.

There are three variables to be considered when determining the manner in which joint movement is affected. They are pain, muscle spasm and physical resistance. It is important to realize that each of these factors, when present, may follow one of many different patterns. Pain, for example, may be present only when joint movement is stretched to the limit of the range; or the opposite may be the case, the joint being painful when it is at rest. It may vary in other ways too; if pain starts early in a range of movement, it does not always worsen in the same pattern when the joint is moved further. For example, the pain felt during movement may be quite moderate until nearing the limit of the range, when it suddenly increases to become severe. On the other hand, the pain may increase in intensity considerably in the first part of the movement and then maintain a steady degree of pain until the limit of range is reached. Different patterns of behaviour of pain require different treatment techniques.'

When pain appears very early in the range and increases sharply as is usually the case when a headache is coming from the occipito-atlanto-axial (O/C1/C2) joints, treatment pressures must be very carefully measured. Five Grade I pressures are often sufficient to alleviate a severe pain which could equally be exacerbated by more.

This fact is of the utmost importance in the treatment of cervical headaches. Severe headaches are likely to arise from a very irritable joint condition in the upper cervical spine and are commonly overtreated. Inexpeıienced manipulators do not always appreciate how easily a severe headache can be relieved by even a few low grade pressures, for example five Grade I pressures. Such a minimal application of mobilization might have no effect at other vertebral levels but is surprisingly effective at the craniovertebral level. Consequently, too many or too strong pressures (even 10 Grade II) constitute overtreatment at the first session and could result in a serious exacerbation of symptoms.

Where the joint movement is restricted by resistance rather than by pain it should be more firmly treated. This is hardly ever the case in the initial presentation of cervical headaches but could apply towards the end of the course of treatment when the pain has been relieved by means of a regimen of gentle mobilization and no longer constitutes the limiting factor. At this stage the periodicity and intensity will have declined with the increase of pain-free movement of the culpable joint. Grade IV and V techniques should clear the joint to a pain-free and resistance-free full range and the headaches should then abate altogether.

When the third variable, muscle spasm, is encountered it must be noted and used as an assessment factor. If it is less or absent on the following day, it tells one that the treatment is being beneficial. Muscle spasm will often be provoked if the pressures are applied in a sharp or jerky manner and will prevent effective movement being imparted to the joint. One should endeavour to press evenly and gently through the spasm in order to move the joint beneath it.

> 'These tests will provide information about joint disorders which is more valuable than that determined by testing in any other way. Details regarding learning to feel these factors found on joint movement, and a method of recording them diagrammatically for purposes of communication and teaching are explained at length in Appendices I and II (p. 351, *Vertebral Manipulation*).
>
> When testing these movements it is necessary, when abnormality is found, to test the same movement in the intervertebral joints above and below, and in the same joints on the opposite side. The physiotherapist should also make use of his experience to compare what is found on examination against what he feels should be normal.'

Tests for the upper cervical spine

> 'Movements of C1 produced by postero-anterior pressure against the arch of the atlas is tested first with the patient prone resting her forehead on her hands (*see Figure 10.1*, p. 90). The physiotherapist applies pressure to three main points: centrally over the posterior tubercle, laterally behind the occipito-atlantal joint and more laterally where the bony arch of the atlas is freely accessible. Occipito-atlantal movement can also be tested by pressure against the anterior surface of C1 at its lateral limits (*see Figure 10.4*, p. 94).
>
> The main testing pressures for the second cervical vertebra with the patient's head still in the same position are directed postero-anteriorly first against the spinous process (*see Figure 10.1*) and then transversely against the tip of the spinous process (*Figure 8.9*). The patient is then asked to turn her head to one side (say to the left) placing her left hand at the level of her head and her right arm by her side. This position allows her left shoulder to lift slightly taking all strain off the cervical rotation. In this position two tests are carried out. The first is transverse pressure on the tip of the lateral mass of the first cervical vertebra' (*see Figure 10.2*, p. 91).

The main source of very many headaches is to be found by means of this last technique. It must be approached especially gently. In many people pressure here is painful but to varying degrees. The more sensitive to pressure it is the more likely is it to be symptomatic. Dramatic and immediate relief of severe headaches can be achieved by the gentlest disturbance of O/C1 in this direction but disproportionate exacerbation of not only pain but dizziness and nausea are likely

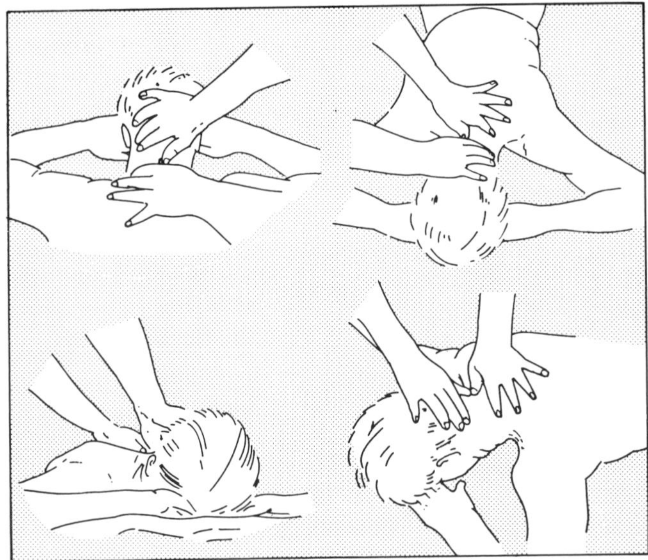

Figure 8.9 Transverse vertebral pressure ←•—

to occur when more than a Grade I pressure, or even too many Grade I pressures are applied initially.

> 'The second is a postero-anterior pressure on the articular pillar of the second cervical vertebra (*Figure 8.10*). It must be remembered that when the patient lies in this position the head, and with it the first cervical vertebra, has rotated to the left; C2 has not moved. Therefore the position of the spinous process of C2 will be the same as it would have been had the head not been rotated. The postero-anterior pressure on the articular pillar of C2 on the right will test the rotation between C1 and C2.'

In the cervical spine it is also possible and useful to carry out antero-posterior pressures against the anterior surface of the spinous processes. The patient lies supine, with her head on a thin pillow rotated very slightly to the right. The therapist stands behind her head, cupping her chin in his right hand. With his left thumb he palpates for the anterior surface of the transverse process of the vertebra to be mobilized. That of C1 and C2 will be palpated anterior to the origin

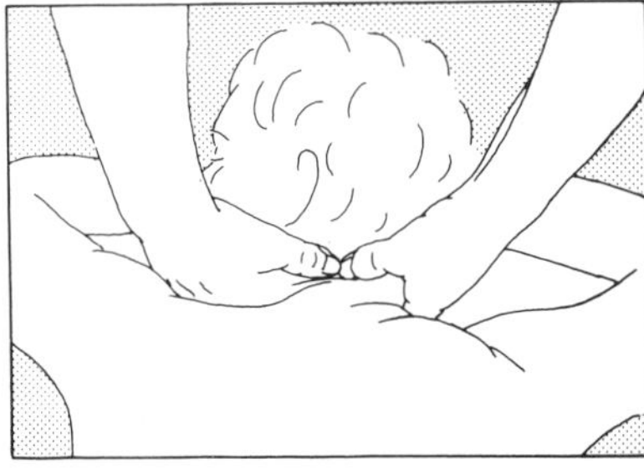

Figure 8.10 Postero-anterior pressure on the articular pillar of C2

of the sternocleidomastoid and those of C3 to C7 posterior to the belly of this muscle. Pressures are exerted in an antero-posterior direction. This palpation technique should not be omitted when the patient indicates parietal pain on the same side. It is also effective, then, as a treatment technique for parietal pain.

Middle and lower cervical spine

'The routine tests in this area include postero-anterior pressures against the spinous process and articular pillar (*Figures 10.1*, p. 90 and *10.3*, p. 93). When testing below C2 the medially directed pressure should routinely be tested (*Figure 8.7b*). The spinous processes of the mid cervical vertebrae are not sufficiently accessible to test with transverse pressure but a similar test can be

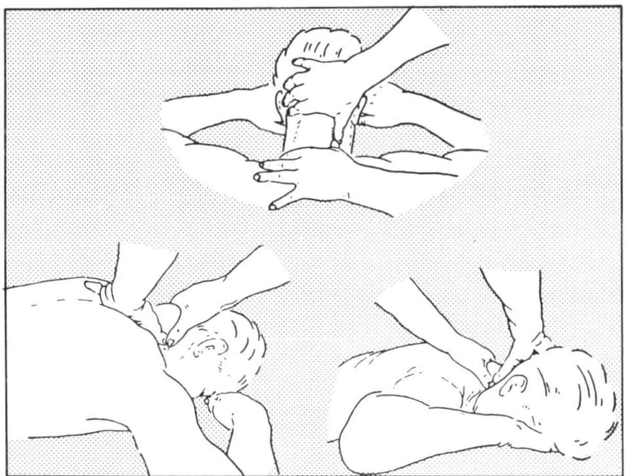

Figure 8.11 Alternative transverse vertebral pressure (C2–C6) ←•—

achieved by pressure against the articular pillar laterally (*Figure 8.11*). In the lower cervical spine transverse pressure against the spinous process can be effected easily. All variations of the directions of the pressures should be assessed if required.'

Temporomandibular joint tests

The temporomandibular joint should not be overlooked when seeking the source of headaches but one should only examine it if there is good reason to suspect that it might be the source of the syndrome. It is my experience that a dormant subsymptomatic temporomandibular joint is best left undisturbed. Severe pain is easily provoked where, undisturbed, it might have remained subsymptomatic.

One should suspect a temporomandibular source in the presence of the following clinical factors:

1. Pain in the lower two-thirds of the trigeminal distribution, e.g. maxillary, paranasal, aural, dental, jaw or cheek pain.
2. Exceptionally severe pain in any of the above areas, particularly when focal structures (ears, nose, teeth, etc.) have been examined and found to be sound.
3. A bizarre and erratic periodicity pattern, impossible to classify in the manner suggested for establishing the TPP (Chapter 7).
4. A pain that had previously been diagnosed as 'tic doloreux' or trigeminal neuralgia but failed to respond to appropriate treatment.

For further information on the temporomandibular joint tests *see* Maitland (1977), Rocabado (1985) and Trott (1986).

Examination of physiological movements

The patient, sitting comfortably, is asked to open her mouth as wide as she is able. She should then close her mouth as hard as she can. With teeth parted she should move her chin to the left and then to the right, then poke it forward and then pull it back again. Any pain felt in the performance of these movements must be reported and recorded, stating range and severity. The smoothness of the movements should also be noted, and the range compared to the contralateral side and to what the therapist thinks would be normal.

Examination of accessory movement

If no pain was felt during the movements, passive overpressure should be given at the end of range, checking for pain. The following tests are then performed, all described for testing the right temporomandibular joint:

Postero-anterior pressure (Figure 8.12). The patient lies prone with her head turned to the right. The therapist stands on the patient's left side facing her head. He places his right thumb, pad facing forward, against the posterior surface of the ascending ramus of the mandible on the right, as close to the joint as possible. Two or three Grade I pressures are then exerted, seeking a pain response. If it is forthcoming one should note the severity and compare it to similar pressures on the contralateral joint.

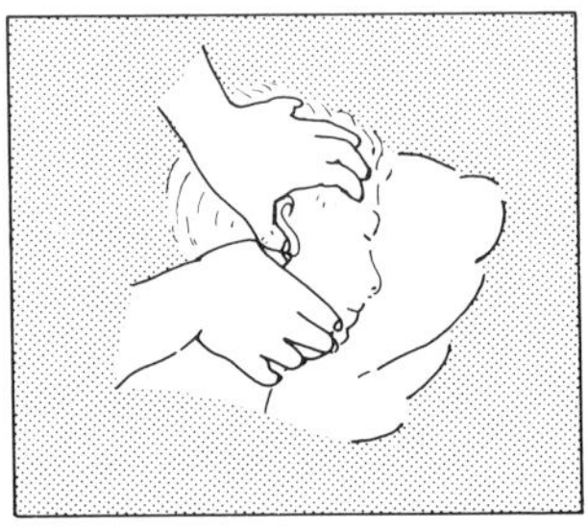

Figure 8.12 Temporomandibular joint; postero-anterior movement

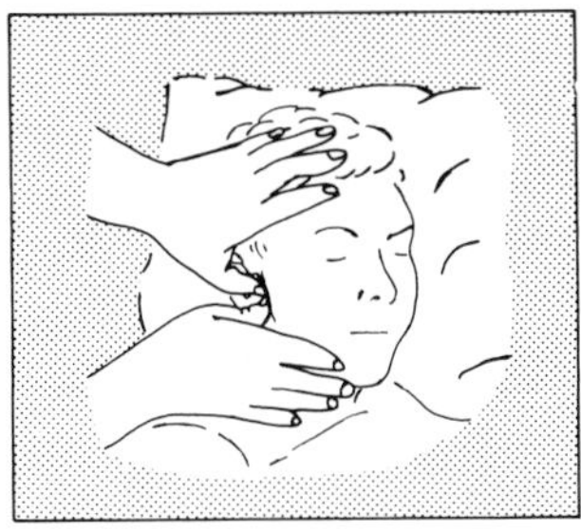

Figure 8.13 Temporomandibular joint: transverse movement medially

Transverse pressure into the joint space (Figure 8.13). The patient and therapist remain in the same positions as in the foregoing test. The therapist leans over the patient's head and asks the patient to open and close her mouth whilst he palpates the joint space. Once he has located it in this way, he asks the patient to hold the mouth open sufficiently for him to be able to insert the tip of his right thumb, pad forward, into the joint space. Two or three Grade I pressures are given and the pain response assessed as before.

Anterolateral pressures. The patient and therapist remain in the same position as for the previous tests and the therapist inserts his right thumb into the patient's right ear, pad forward and palpates the location of the joint while the patient opens and closes her mouth. Once he feels where the movement is taking place he asks her to hold the mouth partially open but relaxed and exerts a couple of laterally directed Grade I pressures and assesses pain response.

Lateral pressures (Figure 8.14) The patient lies supine and the therapist, wearing a glove, inserts his left thumb into the patient's mouth and palpates the temporomandibular joint from the inside, assessing pain response as in the foregoing tests.

If no pain is elicited on any of these test techniques, he should vary his direction and point of contact before using stronger pressure. Once the most painful technique has been found in this manner, the same technique should be used as

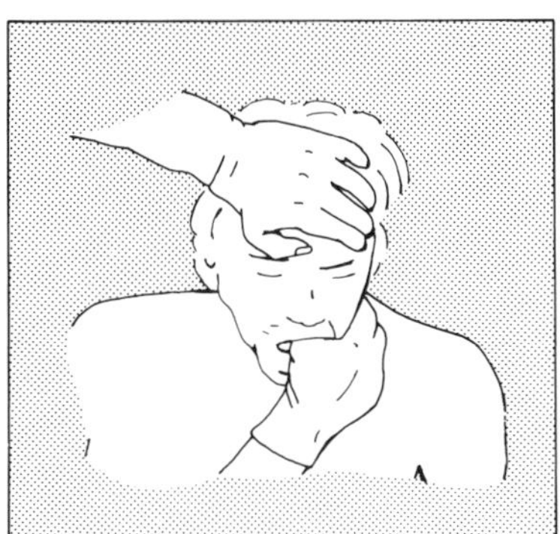

Figure 8.14 Temporomandibular joint: transverse movement laterally

a treatment technique, but not exceeding five Grade I pressures at the first session to avoid the possibility of a bad exacerbation of pain.

Before going on to planning the treatment, X-rays and other test results should be examined and evaluated in terms of the presenting symptoms.

Vertebral artery patency tests must be performed (*see* Chapter 15).

References

Hohl, M. (1964) Normal motions of the upper portion of the cervical spine. *Journal of Bone and Joint Surgery*, **46A** (8), 1777–1779

Maitland, G. D. (1977) Temporomandibular joint. In *Other Joints and Structures: Peripheral Manipulation*, 2nd edn., pp. 318–329. Butterworths, London

Maitland, G. D. (1986) Objective examination. In *Vertebral Manipulation*, 5th edn., pp. 57–94. Butterworths, London

Rocabado, M. ed. (1985) Clinical management of head, neck and TMJ pain and dysfunction. In *Arthrokinematics of the Temporomandibular Joint*. W. B. Saunders, London

Trott, P. H. (1986) Examination of the Temporomandibular Joint. In *Modern Manual Therapy of the Vertebral Column*, ed. G. P. Grieve, Churchill Livingstone, Edinburgh

White, A. A. III and Panjabi, M. M. (1978) The clinical biomechanics of the occipitoatlantoaxial complex. *Orthopaedic Clinics of North America*, **9** (4), 867–878

Further reading

Johnson, P. (1985) Normal temporomandibular joint movements: a pilot study. Proceedings of the 4th Biennial Congress of the Manipulative Therapists Association of Australia, Queensland

Jull, G. (1986) Clinical Observations of upper cervical mobility. In Grieve, G. P. ed. *Modern Manual Therapy of the Vertebral Column*, Churchill Livingstone, Edinburgh

9

Assessment

Assessment begins at first contact with the patient. Even before the subjective examination has begun the experienced therapist has gained an impression: the urgency with which the appointment is requested, perhaps, or the drawn and anxious appearance of the patient when she arrives.

Throughout the subjective questioning this assessment continues. The questions which arise in the examiner's mind are phrased so that the patient understands them, and the patient's responses are considered and interpreted in terms of the headache condition. The answers are evaluated, relevant or useful items are recorded and others discarded. The information so gathered is being processed by the examiner and related to that which he knows from reading and experience.

(In the following examples, * denotes tentative interpretations.)

Miss X phones to make an appointment. She is not able to take up appointments offered within the next few days but would like one next week.
* She is not in extremities of pain.

She arrives for her first appointment and with a brave smile says that she can't go on like this; her headaches seem to be getting worse.
*? A worsening cervical headache, of sufficient severity to seek help.

Area of distribution of pain (*see* p. 89)

For example, the patient indicates a patch of pain in the parietal area only. It is usually right-sided but occasionally left. She experiences no pain in the neck.
* Ipsilateral anteroposterior vertebral pressures on C2 could turn out to be the therapeutic technique (*see* Chapter 11).
* Lesion is probably O/C1 because there is no neck pain.

Periodicity (P)

The periodicity, if clearly established, is more informative and helpful in the reassessment than any other factor. Time should be spent on recording its pattern. In order to gain the maximum useful information from the periodicity factor, the examiner should bear in mind the following framework of common periodicity patterns of headache:

1. *No headache*. There are people who have never experienced a headache. They are the exception.
* This fact can be useful, taking a retrospective history. If a patient says, for certain, that she never knew what a headache was before she was 20, the

examiner should try to find out what it was that happened to her prior to that age. It could have been a whiplash injury, a blow on the head, an inflammatory disease affecting joints, a job involving extremes of neck strain or exceptional emotional stress. Such information could suggest the cause.

2. *Occasional headache.* Most people have an occasional headache and think of it as a normal human condition. They tend to call it a 'normal headache'. If questioned, they usually say that 'occasional' means less often than once a month, that the intensity is mild to moderate and that it abates if they take a simple analgesic.
* I think that the common 'occasional' headache is an early cervical syndrome which is not an irritable condition and is not triggered by trifling daily irritants. If in the retrospective history it emerges that a 'normal' headache began to increase in periodicity and became so frequent that it was present more of the time than it was not, this fact suggests the typically worsening syndrome of the headache of cervical arthrosis.

3. *Violent headache of recent onset and rapid development.*
* Suggestive of intracranial pathology. Do not attempt treatment until this possibility is excluded by a neurologist.

4. *Headache where the onset and duration is secondary to a specific disease.* Its treatment is that of the disease and does not fall within the spectrum that we will be required to treat, e.g. the headache accompanying meningitis and malaria. However, a patient may relate the onset of her chronic headaches to the meningitis she had years ago. The cervical spine could be suffering the mechanical after-effects of a condition which led to stiffness and our treatment could be appropriate.

5. *Episodic headache.* Infrequent headache which comes, lasts for a predictable period of hours or days, then abates completely until the next attack.
* This suggests the vascular migraine (*see* Chapter 4).

6. *Headaches of short duration occurring repeatedly for a period of weeks or days.*
* Think of cluster headache (also vascular).

7. *The headache in which the periodicity advances over the years from the 'normal' headache to frequent to continuous headache.*
* This is almost certain to derive from the cervical spine (*see* Chapter 4).

8. *A combined headache of cervical and vascular source.*
* (*See* Chapters 2 and 4). This can also be identified with the help of periodicity patterns.

Most headaches will fall into these broad patterns of periodicity. There are other rare conditions which could be the cause of the headache, e.g. pituitary tumours or vidian nerve neuralgia and we will certainly not be able to diagnose or to treat them. It is best, if a headache of bizarre behaviour presents, to have it checked out by a medical specialist.

● A periodicity factor of P 5/5 indicates a very irritable condition. Take care not to exacerbate it unnecessarily.

The periodicity pattern of the headache under examination will become the most useful factor in the daily reassessment. When a continuous headache abates for five minutes, it is no longer a P 5/5 but a P 4/5. When a P 4/5 skips a day it has become a P 3/5 and so on.

Intensity of pain (I)

In the advancing cervical syndrome the pain intensity usually increases along with the periodicity.

● The severity of the pain, taken alone, does not indicate a serious pathology. Nor is it, as is often mistakenly thought, diagnostic of a migraine. Cervical headache in the advanced stage manifests with extreme pain.

● The intensity of pain has no bearing on the ease with which it may be relieved by means of the treatment described in this book. It often happens that a pain of maximum intensity (I = 4/5 or I = 5/5) abates after the application of just a few judicial pressures, whereas it has not responded in any way to compound analgesics.

● The decline in average intensity of the daily or continuous pain is also indicative of improvement even when the periodicity does not decrease initially (*see* Chapter 6, case 3).

● The *frequency* of the presence of her *maximum* pain could lessen as treatment continues.

Response to analgesics (R)

The response to analgesics declines as the pain intensity worsens. A pain that abates when a couple of analgesics are taken is not a pain of great intensity.

● A poor or lessening response to first simple, and then compound, analgesics indicates a progressively worsening condition. It also confirms the assessment of the pain intensity.

● It may also be useful in assessing improvement during the course of treatment. If a patient reports that her usual daily headache abated after taking two aspirins, and initially she had said that such a dose had had no or little effect, clearly something has changed for the better.

● The quantity of analgesics habitually taken should also be assessed.

● Overdosage must be noted and will give rise to concern. Many patients will say that they have stopped taking any medication because they themselves have become worried about harmful effects. Some will say that the pills just make them lethargic but do not reduce the pain.

● The patient might say that ergotamine derivative drugs have a better effect than others, and this might indicate that there is a vascular component to the headache. On the other hand, if anti-inflammatory drugs are more helpful, an inflammatory cause should be considered.

• If muscle relaxant drugs have no effect, then the prime cause of the headache is unlikely to be muscle contraction. If tranquillizers and antidepressant drugs do not relieve the headache, then a source other than anxiety or depression should be sought.

• Questioning in this section should, perhaps, also enquire about any other drugs being taken for any other condition. Answers could reveal related or unrelated conditions which could affect the firmness with which the objective examination will be carried out or the choice of technique to be employed in treatment (*see* Chapter 15).

Precipitating factors

A headache which is precipitated or aggravated by movements or sustained postures of the head on the neck will certainly point to a cervical source. But a considerable proportion of cervical headaches are less sensitive to cervical movement and postures than to a variety of other factors, notably emotional stress. The assessment of the sort of stress which brings on the pain will serve to gauge the stage of the arthrotic condition. If it is in the early stage, it will be triggered by major disruption such as the loss of income, a divorce or the overextension involved in reaching a difficult goal or impossible deadline. But in the fully developed or advanced stage of the condition the headache will be triggered by trivial daily irritations like losing one's keys or being late for work. Few people live such tranquil lives that they are not subjected to daily irritations but they do not suffer daily headaches as a result.

Cervical headaches are triggered by a large variety of factors which are often specific, as headache triggers, to a particular subject. A headache which responds to alcohol or chocolate should not, on this evidence alone, be diagnosed as a vascular migraine (*see* Chapter 4).

Associated symptoms

Contrary to that which is stated in much of the literature, cervical headaches *are* accompanied by many symptoms other than pain, e.g. visual and aural disturbances, globulus hystericus, epigastric pain, nausea and vomiting and also dizziness. These can also appear as precursors of the headache, although it is more usual, in the cervical headache, that they appear when the headache reaches a high pain intensity.

• When a prodrome of clearly defined visual patterns is described, e.g. sensory hallucinations, visions, scintillating scotomata, fortification spectra and the diffuse autonomic disturbances as described by many writers (and sufferers), the probability is that the subject is suffering from classic migraine (Sacks, 1973).

• Autonomic disturbances which accompany cervical headaches are more commonly spots or moving flashes of light, visual blurring and occasionally ptosis or partial loss or distortion of vision. Loss of distance judgement and photophobia are also common.

• Tinnitus in the form of ringing, humming, or buzzing is very common. Dizziness may be present to the extent that the patient appears to be ataxic.

Nausea and vomiting are common, as is epigastric pain. Many patients, though, say that they associate the epigastric pain with the drugs they take.

● Subjective reports of marked dizziness should warn one against using strong manipulative techniques, or even techniques involving rotation.

Previous investigations, tentative diagnoses, treatment and the response to the treatment

This information can be informative.

● If a severe syndrome has not been neurologically investigated, it is wise to request such tests.

● If migraine-specific treatment had no effect, there is probably no vascular component.

● If a biomechanical procedure applied to the neck (e.g. chiropractic manipulation) had a beneficial effect, the headache is likely to be of cervical articular origin.

● If it is reported that a course of physiotherapy had not been of any benefit, ask what modalities were employed. If the physiotherapy had been the treatment of muscle spasm, it is probable that manipulative treatment will be more successful.

● The number of specialists consulted and failed treatments listed are an indication of the disruptive effect that the headache has had on the life of the patient and her family. It also rules out the probability of other or morbid pathology and this information usually confirms a diagnosis of headache of cervical arthrosis.

● Before proceeding to the objective examination the present intensity of pain (or nausea or dizziness) should be assessed and the therapist will then decide whether to carry out the full objective examination or, if these factors are severe, to use some form of palliative treatment and delay the objective examination until the following day.

Reference

Sacks, O., ed. (1973) *Migraine. The Evolution of a Common Disorder*. Faber and Faber, London

10

Technique

All of the cervical mobilizing and manipulative techniques described by Maitland in *Vertebral Manipulation* could be useful in the treatment of headaches at some stage of the course of treatment. But unless one is very specific in the selection of a technique for a particular pain, and proves its effectiveness by means of careful assessment, one could employ them all and still have no effect upon the headache.

Selection of effective technique

Guide

I believe that the upper cervical spine is the primary source of cervical pain that can be referred to the head. It may often seem that headache is coming from C7, or even from the thoracic spine, because manipulative treatment carried out at these levels is at times found to relieve it. But I think that the lower levels are not a primary but a secondary source and serve to aggravate or perpetuate a headache arising from the upper cervical spine. The syndrome will not be completely cleared until the primary and the secondary sources have been adequately dealt with.

Many writers put forward quite distinct patterns of pain referral from pain sources which fall within their own field of expertise. Such patterns are undoubtedly helpful in locating the lesion, be they cerebral tumours or vascular lesions. However, it should be realized that such patterns are merely a guide and that pain in any area of the head can arise from any one of many sources. The pain of cervical spondylosis can refer to any part of the head and simulate pain arising elsewhere. For example, it is stated by more than one authority that a pain perceived as a tight band around the head indicates a psychogenic condition. But very many such pains can be cleared by means of a simple mobilization of the upper cervical spine, suggesting that they had been of organic origin. *Table 10.1* presents a guide to help therapists locate the cervical articulation causing pain in different parts of the head and the technique which is most likely to succeed in relieving it.

Table 10.1 serves as a guide only and any cervical technique may be tried and might, upon evaluation, prove to be effective in the relief of any of the pains listed in the Table. Each of the techniques has not been adequately evaluated if the direction of pressure and the point of contact has not been varied.

Table 10.1 Guide to locating and techniques for relieving cervical articulation causing pain

Area of pain	*Joint responsible*	*Effective technique*
Vertex	Occipito-atlantal	Central postero-anterior vertebral pressure on C1
Frontal, peri-orbital or temporal	Occipito-atlantal	Transverse vertebral pressures on C1 on the side of pain
Occipital and supra- or retro-orbital	Atlanto-axial or C2/C3	Postero-anterior unilateral pressure on C2 on the side of pain with head straight or rotated to the pain side
Parietal	Occipito-atlantal or atlanto-axial	Antero-posterior unilateral vertebral pressure on C1 or C2 on the pain side
Facial, aural, nasal, tooth or gum	Temporomandibular joint or O/C1	Try all temporomandibular techniques and transverse pressure on C1 on the side of pain
Neck pain and associated eye symptoms	C3	Central and unilateral postero-anterior pressure or anteroposterior pressures

It is recommended that those readers who are not proficient in Maitland's techniques should study these from his book (*Vertebral Manipulation*, 5th edn., Chapters 5, 6, 9) and practise them with the help of a colleague who is.

The author wishes to emphasize certain passages from Maitland's book and reproduces them here for the convenience of the reader:

> 'To produce movement of a joint in any one direction, it is easier to gain the fullest movement, with least effort for the physiotherapist and without strain to the patient, if this joint is positioned approximately in the midposition of all its other ranges.
>
> Techniques which involve pressure against some part of the vertebra require special care. The thumbs or the hands are only the medium through which the physiotherapist's body weight is transmitted to the vertebra to produce movement. If the intrinsic muscles of the hand are used to produce the pressure, the technique will immediately become uncomfortable to both patient and physiotherapist, the hands will become tense and all possibility of 'feeling' the movement will be lost. A study of the diagrams will show how the shoulders are positioned above or behind the hands, and how the joints from the shoulders downwards act as a series of springs. Every effort should be made at the beginning to observe these points.
>
> The starting positions are also important as they allow the patient to relax completely and the physiotherapist to work effectively with the minimum of effort. Relaxation of the physiotherapist's hands is essential, for it is impossible to feel through hands which are tense.'

Grades of mobilization

All the techniques to be described may be applied in any of four grades.

> 'Grade I is a tiny amplitude movement near the starting position of the range.

Grade II is a large amplitude movement which carries well into the range. It can occupy any part of the range but does not reach the limit of the range.
Grade III is also a large amplitude movement but one which reaches the limit of range or the limiting resistance.
Grade IV is a tiny amplitude movement at the limit of the range. The arrows, marked for each of the four grades, depict the amplitude of each of the movements and the position they occupy in the range.'

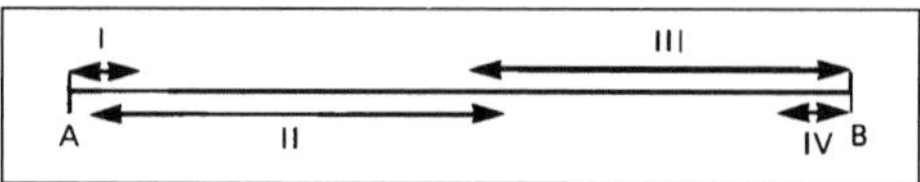

The following techniques are described by Maitland (1986) but transcribed here and adapted so as to apply specifically to the symptom of headache.

Postero-anterior central vertebral pressure on C1 (*Figure 10.1*)

The patient lies face down with her head extending slightly over the end of the couch. The therapist stands facing the crown of the patient's head. He asks the patient to tuck in her chin so that her forehead rests on the couch and to accept the support of the therapist's thigh and to press gently against it so as to allow for

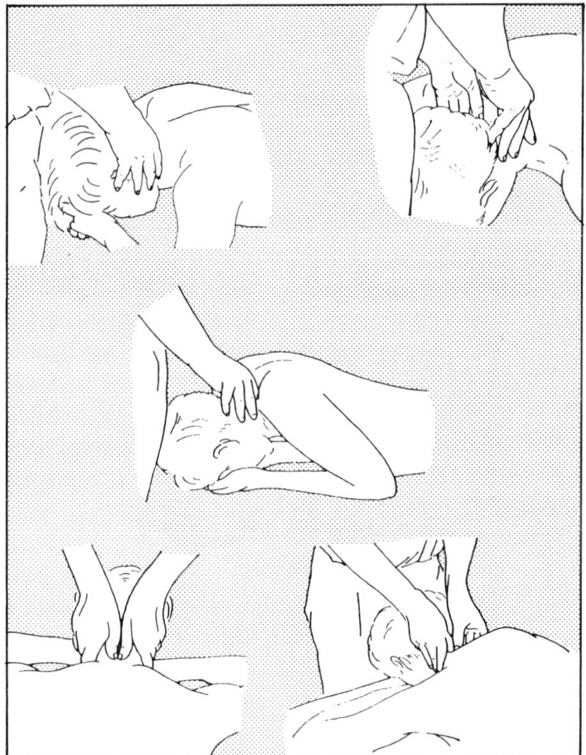

Figure 10.1 Postero-anterior central vertebral pressure on C1

relaxation of her (the patient's) upper cervical ligaments. Maintaining this support, the therapist leans over the patient and places his two thumbs, either adjacent and back to back or one reinforcing the other, on the spinous process of C2. He slides them down the superior surface of this spinous process until he feels the posterior surface of the arch of the atlas, where the tubercle can often be felt. This is midway between the inferior surface of the base of the occiput and the spinous process of C2. In some cases where the ligamentum nuchae is well developed it is not possible to make bony contact with the arch of the atlas and the required pressure should then be determined by the pain response. If this technique affects the source of the headache it will be extremely painful. The therapist should slowly direct his pressure through the resistant ligaments until a pain response is elicited. He should then apply five equal pressures at this same strength and then reassess the symptoms.

Because of the tight structures overlying this joint the pressure required to elicit a response is sometimes quite considerable. It would not be effective to apply grades of movement before the pain response is elicited but one should judge the commencement of pain with the utmost of care and apply grades from this point. Grade I pressures should just initiate the pain response with each pressure.

Transverse vertebral pressure against the tip of the transverse process of C1 (—•→) (*Figure 10.2*)

(For a left-sided pain)

The patient lies prone with her head rotated to the left. Her left hand is placed in front of her face and the right arm lies at her right side. The therapist stands in front of the patient facing her head. He inserts his left thumb tip, pad facing forward, into the angle formed between the ascending ramus of the left mandible and the anterior surface of the mastoid process. At a point roughly midway between the tip of the mastoid process and the angle of the mandible he sinks the thumb tip in until he feels bony contact. Should there be a sharp pain response before he is conscious of the bony contact, he should judge the depth at which this occurred and measure Grade I pressures from this point.

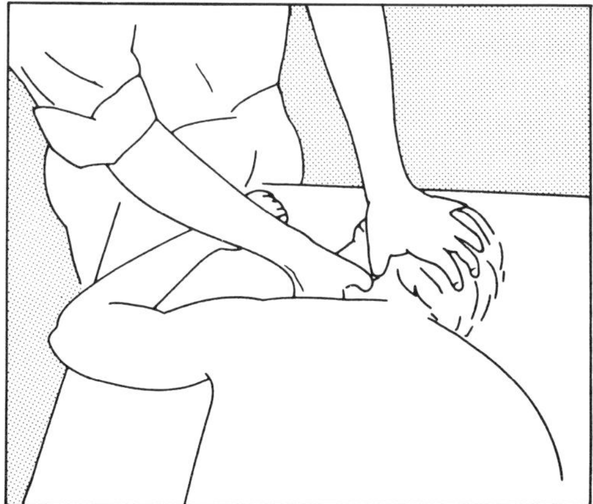

Figure 10.2 Transverse vertebral pressure —•→

If there is no pain response he might go a little deeper and then, if it is still not painful, he should move his point of contact upwards or downwards within that angle, probing gently for a painful response, and also vary the direction of the pressures. It is most often to be found high towards the apex of the mandibular/mastoid angle.

This is often a dormant source of pain and therefore tender to pressure even if it is not the source of the current symptoms. One should compare it with the pain elicited with the same pressure on the contralateral side and if it is markedly more painful it is probable that it is the source of the ipsilateral pain.

An alternative position for the patient with restricted rotation is that of side lying with the head resting on a pillow.

If the mandibular/mastoid angle is very close, place a rolled up towel under the patient's neck to open it up and palpate again. As it is essential to use the tip of the thumb, the thumbnail should be filed very short.

Method

Pressures should be directed transversely through the head towards the opposite ear. It is not possible to use this technique effectively if the thumbnail protrudes beyond the tip. The direction may be varied in accordance with the findings on palpation, using the most painful direction of movement. The grade should be determined not by the sense of movement perceived by the therapist as is the case in mobilizing techniques used for other conditions, but by the pain response. This can be reliably determined by watching the flicker of the patient's eye at the onset of each pressure. If, at a certain pressure or grade the eye remains impassive, that grade will not be effective. More than the merest flicker of the eye, however, indicates too strong a grade and one should fall back to a lighter grade.

When this technique is being used for the first time on a patient, one should never exceed five Grade I pressures, measured as described above. This is perhaps the joint in the body most easily and therefore most commonly overtreated. It is not usually appreciated how dramatically just a few of the gentlest possible pressures can relieve the most stubborn and severe headache. Treatment at this joint should only be increased when successive mobilizing sessions have gained improvement without negative side-effects or aggravation of the headache. In such cases the treatment dose could be increased to 20 Grade IV pressures and more. When the periodicity and/or intensity of the headache syndrome has markedly declined but no further improvement is achieved by repeated applications of Grade IV, a Grade V manipulative technique effective at the O/C1 level may clear the joint and the symptoms should abate altogether. This should only be done if there are no contraindications to this procedure (*see* Chapter 15).

Postero-anterior unilateral vertebral pressure on C2 (•⌐↓)

(*Figure 10.3*)

(For a right-sided pain)

The patient lies prone with her forehead cupped in the palms of her hands. The therapist stands facing the crown of her head and leans over the patient so that

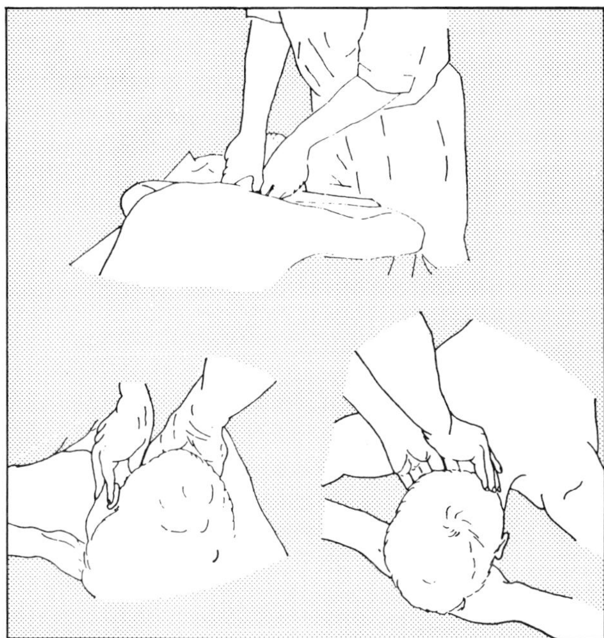

Figure 10.3 Postero-anterior unilateral vertebral pressure •┐

his shoulders are above the joint to be treated. He places his two thumbs on the posterior surface of the spinous process of the second cervical vertebra, nail to nail or one superior and the other inferior. Holding his thumbs thus he palpates with his fingers, the lateral extent of the articular pillar at this level. Holding his right forefinger against the lateral surface of the transverse process of C2, which has been localized in this manner, he moves his thumb towards the right index finger until they come to rest on the posterior surface of the articular pillar at level C2.

Method

Pressure should be directed straight downwards in the chosen grade, determined by the pain response as described in the foregoing technique. As this joint is slightly less resentful of early movement, initial treatment could go to 10 Grade II pressures.

In seeking the pain response one might vary the point of contact from the lateral edge of C2 along the posterior surface as far as the lateral border of the spinous process. The direction should also be varied at each point of contact to incline towards the patient's head, towards her feet, medially and laterally before one would exclude that movement as the painful one. This technique will cause relative movement between C2 and C3.

The same technique done with the patient's head turned slightly to the right, thumbs in the same position as described above, will cause movement between C1 and C2.

Postero-anterior unilateral pressure on C1 (•⅂↓)

With the patient and the therapist in the same positions as for the technique postero-anterior central pressure on C1, the therapist palpates along the nuchal line, exerting gentle pressures as he moves laterally until he feels the occipito-atlantal articulation. He exerts, as with other trial techniques, Grade I pressures seeking a pain response and imparts no more than five Grade I pressures at this stage until symptoms have been reassessed on the following day.

Anteroposterior unilateral vertebral pressure (*Figure 10.4*)

(Performed on the right for right-sided parietal pain)

The patient lies supine with her head resting on the therapist's flexed left knee which is placed on the couch. The therapist stands by her head and holds the patient's head in his left hand and forearm, rotating it slightly to the left. He then palpates the anterior surface of the transverse process of C2 with his right thumb, using the pad.

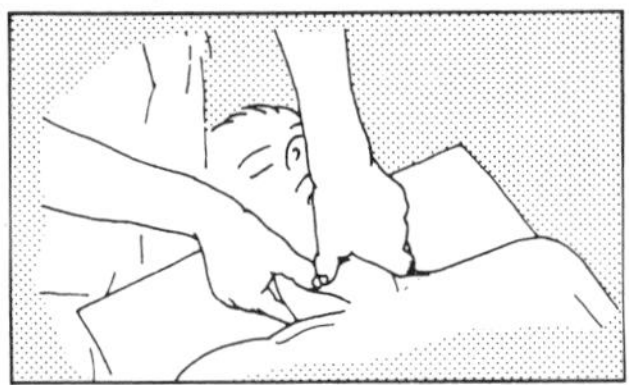

Figure 10.4 Unilateral anteroposterior vertebral pressure •_↑

Method

Anteroposterior pressures are applied at the point of contact and in the direction which elicits a sharp pain response, judging the grade by means of the onset of the pain response as indicated by the flicker of the patient's eye. Five to ten pressures can be given at the first treatment.

Temporomandibular joint techniques

(Used on the side of pain)

The techniques described in Chapter 8 for palpating the temporomandibular joint for the source of pain are used as treatment techniques. As the pain-causing condition of this joint is often extremely irritable, it should be approached initially with the greatest care in order not to subject the patient to a violent exacerbation of pain. Having established the painful direction of movement and the depth of range at which the pain comes in, no more than five Grade I pressures should be exerted at this point.

The techniques described here will deal with the majority of headaches.

Practical applications

When the head pain is localized to one area in the head, say the vertex, and it is present when treatment is commenced, record this before applying the trial technique and try to effect a change with the technique before going on to another.

For example:

Now c/o* localized vertex pain, moderate intensity
o/e* central postero-anterior pressure painful to Grade I pressure.

Treatment	*Immediate response*
Central postero-anterior vertebral pressure Grade I × 5 pressures	Vertex pain less intense
Repeat above technique	Vertex pain gone

No more mobilization should be aimed at treating that pain. But if there was, and still is another pain area, e.g. left temporal pain, another technique should be applied attempting to get rid of that, thus:

Now c/o* left temporal pain, mild intensity
o/e* transverse pressure, Grade I on C1–sharp pain

Treatment	*Immediate response*
C1 Grade I × 5 transverse pressures towards the right	Left temporal pain gone

The physiotherapist should then establish whether the patient has any or no pain anywhere in the head and, if none, no more mobilization should be given on that day. If yet another area of pain is present it should be treated with an appropriate technique as before.

The foregoing serves to demonstrate how techniques should be applied specifically in an attempt to relieve a specific pain and not in a haphazard manner hoping that one or other technique is effective. Overtreatment not only confuses assessment but exposes the patient to a bad exacerbation.

The most reliable assessment parameter for use in evaluating headache techniques is an immediate change in the pain following the application of a technique. This change may be either of the following. The pain:

has shifted
is less intense
has become more diffuse
has localized
has intensified
has gone.

* c/o, patient complains of; o/e, objective examination.

Any of the above signifies a positive response to a technique and that technique should be pursued as described in Chapter 11.

Reference

Maitland, G. D., ed. (1986) *Vertebral Manipulation*, 5th edn. Butterworth, London

11

Treatment and progression of treatment

When the subjective and physical examinations have been completed and the initial assessment made, treatment, guided by continuous reassessment, is commenced.

Although the patient's usual pain pattern will already have been recorded, the patient should be asked, immediately prior to the application of the first technique:

'Do you feel any pain in the head now?' If so
'Where do you feel it?' and
'How severe is it?' and
'Do you feel any sensation other than pain?'

This information should be recorded under the word NOW on the chart and then proceed as follows. The selection of techniques is made according to the method taught by Maitland (1986) whereby the usefulness of each technique is evaluated during a process of ongoing assessment (*see* Chapter 4). Although this method decides the actual technique used, the following list serves as a guide as to which technique to try first:

1. *Isolated head pain*: transverse pressures on C1 on the side of pain. Remember to angle the pressures and to vary the point of thumb contact in order not to miss the painful direction of accessory movement.
2. *Occipital pain*: unilateral postero-anterior vertebral pressure on C2 on the side of pain. If the pain is bilateral, treat both sides.
3. *Vertex pain and/or pressure*: central postero-anterior vertebral pressures on C1.
4. *Parietal pain*: unilateral antero-posterior pressure on the side of pain, C1 and C2. If the pain is bilateral, treat both sides.
5. *Headache with associated neck or throat pain*. Start with the appropriate technique for pain in the head as suggested above and also attend to painful synovial articulations further down in the cervical spine, particularly C3 and C7.

Let us say that the patient is complaining of a long-standing and continuous pain above the right eye and that it is present at the time of first treatment, before the application of the first trial technique. It is of moderate intensity and she also feels nauseous. Record thus:

Now: Pain over R eye
Moderate intensity
Nausea

Treatment Transverse vertebral pressure on C1, directed from right to left (←• C1)

Grade I × 5 pressures // Result of this technique.

The result could have been:

Favourable	*Unfavourable*
Pain has gone	Pain is unchanged
Pain has lessened	Pain has worsened
Pain has shifted	Nausea is unchanging
Pain has become more diffuse	Nausea has worsened
Pain has become more localized	
Nausea has gone	
Nausea has lessened	

If it seems from the foregoing subjective examination that the condition is an irritable one, stop today's treatment here and ask the patient to come again on the following day. Warn her that she might experience an exacerbation of symptoms. Explain to her that, if she does, it is not an unfavourable reaction and that it is not to be expected after subsequent treatments. She should not be alarmed even if she experiences a headache very much worse than is usual for her, but must report it to the therapist.

Tell her, too, that there may be a change in the pattern of her headache as she has come to know it and as she has described it in the subjective examination. She should monitor the behaviour of the pain and other symptoms for the 24 hours after the treatment and report changes, even if they seem to her to be insignificant. If the headache which was there just prior to the treatment had gone away as a result of treatment, it is important for her to note the length of the pain-free period and report it the following day. Alternatively, if it had not gone away as a result of the treatment, she should notice whether it went away at all during the ensuing 24 hours and for how long it stayed away. If it had become worse after treatment, she should be able to tell on the following day for how long it had remained worse, and whether it then settled to its previous level or went away.

If there is reason to think that it was an irritable condition and the first trial technique resulted in a slight decrease in the pain, that technique should be repeated using only five pressures before assessing the result in the same way as before, judging whether there is a further decrease or whether the pain has gone.

If there was no change in the symptoms after the first technique and the condition does not seem to be irritable, another technique should be tried, say unilateral postero-anterior vertebral pressures on the occipito-atlantal joint on the right, Grade I × 5 pressures and reassess.

If there had been positive movement signs which were elicited during the objective examination, one would need to reassess these and record the result before the patient goes home.

After the mobilization and reassessment, the therapist may use any other appropriate modality but not exercise or massage at this stage.

D + 1

On the second day (D + 1) the behaviour of the pain and nausea must be assessed again for the period between the previous day's treatment and this visit, and compared with the same period over the previous 24 hours.

Movement signs should be checked and compared with the recording of the previous day, noting improvement. The result is recorded. Palpation tests of intervertebral movement should be reassessed and compared with those of the previous day and any change recorded. One might perceive:

Less stiffness
Less pain reported on the same grade of pressure
Less feeling of thickness or oedema

If the assessment reflects improvement even if it is only marginal, the previous day's treatment should be repeated exactly but giving a slightly bigger 'dose', which means a small increase in grade of pressure and number of pressures. For example:

Treatment Transverse vertebral pressures on C1 from right to left.
Grade I × 10 pressures or Grade I+ × 10 (←• C1).

If the assessment reveals an exacerbation, the previous day's treatment should be repeated exactly but with a slight decrease in dosage or kept the same. For example:

Treatment Transverse vertebral pressure on C1 from the right to left.
Grade I × 5 pressures.

If the assessment shows that the pain worsened as a result of the previous day's treatment, remained worse and is still worse when she arrives for her second treatment, apply some form of palliative treatment and try to think why the treatment could have had an unfavourable effect

OR

try an indirect technique, e.g. apply the technique to the contralateral joint

OR

try a passive physiological movement technique, e.g. rotation gently, Grade II –

OR

try gentle manual traction sustained for half a minute and reassess.

Try to relieve the pain that is present but do not overtreat as the poor reaction was most likely as a result of overtreatment yesterday.

Reassess on the following day. Exacerbation in chronic headache cases can be extremely severe, and so it is important to warn the patient of the possibility and to reassure her if it should happen. The therapist should not be alarmed if the patient telephones him at some time after a treatment to say that she is experiencing the worst headache she has ever had. She should be reassured and told to take whatever she usually takes for pain and to rest with a cold compress on the treatment area, or warmth if she cannot tolerate cold. She should return the following day. Even when the first treatment comprises 5 × Grade I pressures, about 20% of those treated could be expected to flare up. Most of these will experience an improvement after the flare up settles down. If the pain remains worse after the second day, consult with the patient's doctor and tell him that she is responding unfavourably.

D + 2

If there are signs of improvement, repeat the previous day's treatment and if there has been no exacerbation the dosage may be fairly rapidly increased to Grades II, III and IV, and up to 20 such pressures on subsequent days during which the ongoing reassessment continues, guiding the technique. By now daily improvement should become evident.

If improvement slows down or stops, alternative techniques must be evaluated and used. Perhaps adjacent joints should be included in the treatment or the direction of movement in the treatment techniques should be varied.

Treatment progress

If the pain had been present continuously or daily (P = 5/5 or 4/5), treat daily until the pain skips a day. Then treat every second day.

At this stage it will not matter if a weekend intervenes, but the patient must be asked to note the behaviour of symptoms for the 24 hours after the Friday treatment and report on Monday. Some patients would need to jot it all down or else the assessment of the Friday's treatment could be lost. It is, however, important to see the patient on the day following the first treatment, and if this was on Friday they should report on Saturday even if it is telephoned in. They will at that stage still be inexperienced at monitoring their symptoms and by Monday will have forgotten important detail.

When the pain skips more than a day, a few days may be skipped between treatments in order to see how long the remission is lasting.

When the symptoms skip several days, the next appointment should be booked for a week's time. If there had been no headache during that week, treat as on the previous visit, perhaps with a larger dose. There will still be joint signs of tenderness on passive movement but only at a stronger grade. Then one should see the patient after two weeks and reassess.

If there has been no headache for two weeks, a last treatment of Grade IV pressures should be given and the patient discharged PRN (pro re nata) which means that she need not attend for treatment until she has her next headache. She should telephone whenever that might be and make another appointment. At that appointment the periodicity should be reassessed and also the total pain pattern (TPP) in order to judge improvement in the syndrome since commencement of treatment.

For management after this stage see Chapter 13 on post-discharge management.

Reference

Maitland, G. D. (1986) *Vertebral Manipulation*, 5th edn., Chapter 7. Butterworths, London.

12

Difficult cases

There will be, in any disorder, a variable response to the same treatment. Over 70% of the true cervical headaches can be expected to respond well to treatment by mobilization as described in this book (Edeling, 1974, 1986) and the remaining percentage will be slow responders, poor responders and non-responders. On first examination these may not seem to differ clinically from those which will respond well (*see* more detailed grouping in Chapter 13).

Because the large majority of chronic non-vascular headaches clear up so easily and often dramatically when the offending joints are mobilized, the therapist may be inclined, when slow or poor response is encountered, to give up too soon. However, in consideration of the history of the chronic headache sufferer (Edeling, 1986), the practitioner would be reluctant to abandon a case where all previous treatment had been unsuccessful and the patient's health is at risk from the overuse of drugs. The therapist has often been the last port of call.

This book deals in detail with the examination and treatment of the pain which emanates from cervical joints, but if this fails attention should be focused on disorders of other systems which could be causing or contributing to the chronic headache. If the therapist decides to pursue further investigation and other approaches, and the patient is willing, the following route is suggested.

Reassessment in more depth

Reconsider the diagnosis

Consider whether the joints are unresponsive to mobilization because of the presence of primary osteoarthritis. An anti-inflammatory drug would be more effective in this case, either supplementing or replacing treatment by mobilization.

Determine whether there could be an element of *migraine*. Chronic headache often presents with a dual pathology where the cervical and vascular components are both operative (*see* Chapter 2). The mechanical disorder of the intervertebral joints in close proximity to the vertebral artery could be triggering a vascular headache by means of a mechanism yet to be agreed upon. If this is the case, mobilization of the offending joints will reduce the occurrence of the migraine and the patient should be advised to seek medication for the migraine from her medical doctor.

Re-examine the cervical joint source

Before examining other structures the *cervical joint source* should be re-examined in more depth. A searching, probing reassessment should be carried out to determine whether there has been *some* or *no* response. Covert response which might have gone unnoticed by therapist and patient alike could mean that this is a slow responder and that the treatment should be intensified or prolonged. This reassessment should cover the following aspects:

Periodicity (P)

Assess for a minor decline in the periodicity. A rapid decline in the periodicity is readily noticed and reported by the patient but when the decline is gradual it is sometimes overlooked. Many patients are more inclined to focus on the pain that remains and not on that which is no more. The reader will be familiar with the patient who had been in constant pain for a prolonged period and whose pain had abated after yesterday's treatment and remained absent for a significant period, who reports on the following day that there is no improvement and that the pain is as bad as ever. Careful questioning is required in order to glean the necessary truth. It can be achieved by saying to the patient who reports no change:

> 'Do you remember that yesterday you told me (reading from the therapist's notes) that your forehead pain, although it was sometimes severe and sometimes mild, was never gone? That it had been continuous for the past many months?' (Patient agrees.)
> 'Before you lay down on the couch for the first treatment, the pain was there, in the forehead as usual and of a moderate intensity.' (Patient agrees.)
> 'After I mobilized some very tender joints in your neck, you sat up and said that the pain had gone. You left here with no pain. When did you become aware of that pain again?' (Patient says by the time she got home or at bedtime or whenever.)

She should be made to understand that this is what is important to know and that she should report the length of subsequent remissions and begin to judge, over the course of treatment and after discharge, by how much the periodicity has declined. Patients forget pain and especially if the decline in its presence is gradual they don't realize how much better they are until the therapist reminds them of how they suffered before. In some cases it is useful to employ the concept of a graphic depiction of the 'quantity' of pain over time – quantity being the sum of pain intensity and the frequency of its presence (*see Figures 12.1* and *12.2*)

The most difficult cases to assess are those with a low or erratic pain periodicity. The periodicity factor is the most useful parameter for assessment of progress (*see* Chapter 7).

P = 5/5 Continuous pain
P = 4/5 Pain present every day but not continuous
P = 3/5 Pain present on 2 or 3 days per week
P = 2/5 Pain present on 2 or 3 days per month
P = 1/5 Pain present once a month or less

In the case of P = 5/5, response is promptly assessable. If a pain which had been continuous for any length of time prior to the application of a treatment technique

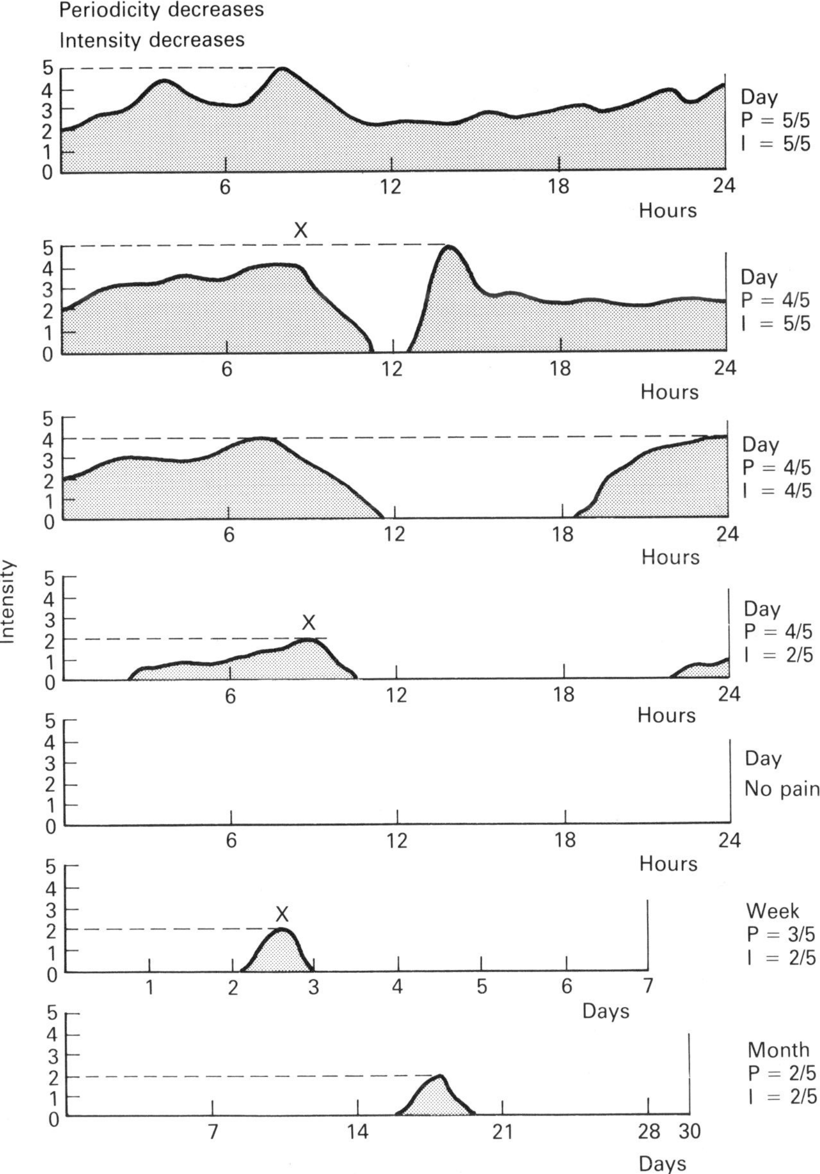

Figure 12.1 Assessment of pain: X indicates a treatment session

abates for even a short spell it is no longer continuous and the therapist can expect that progressively longer periods of remission will follow after subsequent use of the same technique. Similarly, if a P = 4/5 headache skips a day it becomes P = 3/5 and when it skips a week it becomes P = 2/5 and when it skips a month it is P = 1/5. This is the progress to be expected in successful treatment of the cervical headache condition.

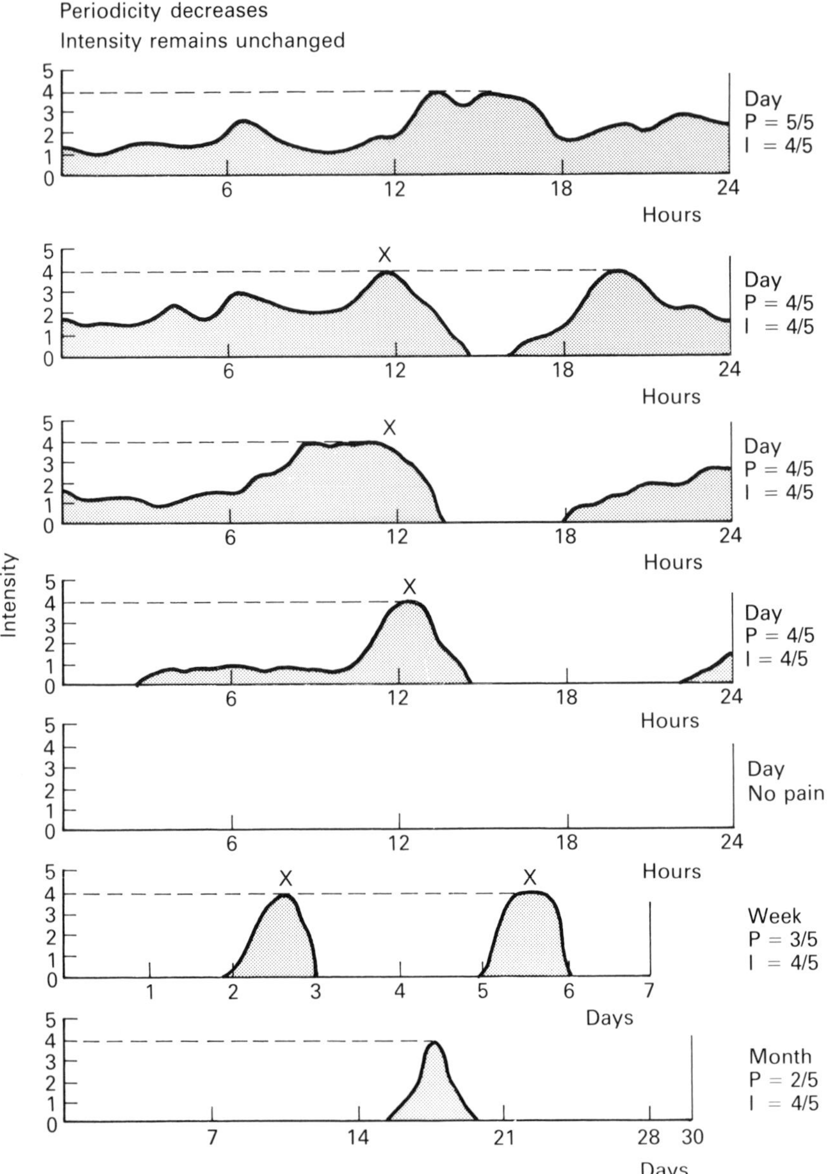

Figure 12.2 Assessment of pain: X indicates a treatment session

However, if the periodicity is irregular, this assessment is complicated because it is not possible to know whether or not these unpredictable remissions are as a result of treatment. In such cases it is necessary to establish with the patient what is the *longest period* that she can expect to be without headache. Help her by bracketing, e.g.: 'Could you go a whole month without a headache? No? A week? Yes. Two weeks? Maybe. Three? No.' In this case we could only claim to have improved the condition if more than three weeks elapse between headaches and then continue until more than a month passes with no pain. By this time one can expect diminished pain intensity and improved response to analgesics, resulting in a total pain pattern (TPP; *see* Chapter 7) consisting of:

P = 1/5
I = 1/5 or 2/5
R = 1/5 or 2/5
TPP = 3/15 or 5/15

which is an acceptable condition, whereas it was, initially, say:

P = 2/5 or 3/5
I = 4/5
R = 4/5
TPP = 10/15 or 11/15

The severity of the initial condition would have required a lot more analgesics because:

- The headaches were present more frequently.
- The greater pain intensity would oblige the use of an analgesic whereas she can cope without pain pills when the intensity of pain is less.
- The pain would abate with a simple analgesic where a more severe pain would require compound analgesics.

Most people experience mild to moderate headache on occasion which abates with a simple analgesic and this is so common that it is called a 'normal headache' (*see* Chapter 2) for which treatment is not sought.

When the patient arrives at the first visit without pain and on questioning it is found that the periodicity pattern is erratic, it will save time and frustration to follow one or other of the following courses:

1. Record a complete subjective and objective examination. Using *Table 10.1* as a guide, palpate the suspect joints using the technique suggested in the Table and, if tender, mobilize accordingly. (It is not necessary to use the very gentle pressures as described elsewhere in this book for the initial treatment as these infrequent headaches are not likely to exacerbate from strong treatment as are the high periodicity ones.)
   Reassess objective signs if present.
   Repeat the treatment for five days. Then stop treatment and ask the patient to report the onset of the next headache, let it run its course and report when it has gone again. From this report one might be able to assess:
   (a) A longer remission than was initially recorded.
   (b) Lessening of overall pain intensity during this bout.
   (c) Better response to analgesics than before.
   (d) A shorter duration of the episode.

If so, then another course of five treatments should be given as before and then stopped to be reassessed when the next bout occurs. This process should be repeated as often as is required and one would hope to achieve an ever lengthening remission period until the headache abates altogether or becomes acceptable to the patient at a TPP of 3/15 or less. At this stage she would no longer need regular treatment but should be told to report back for more treatment if ever the syndrome seems to be escalating again.

OR

2. The patient could be asked to attend for treatment on the day of her next headache. It would be wise to have done the first assessment on the day of initial attendance when the time had been booked so that when she needs to come at short notice it will be easier to fit her in.
   The headache which is then present is assessed and treated, evaluating techniques as in Chapter 10. One should aim to shift, reduce or abate the headache and record the technique which has done so. This technique should be aggressively pursued, repeating and strengthening it until the headaches are gone. The patient is then asked to report for treatment each time it recurs until there is sufficient reduction in the syndrome.

Intensity (I)

Reassess for a decline in the pattern of pain intensity. It happens, not infrequently, that during the course of treatment of a slow responder that the patient says the headache is still there all the time. One could then ask her: 'Are you no better than before we started this treatment?' and she may answer: 'Oh yes, I'm much better'. Asked: 'In what way?' she may say: 'My headaches are no longer so severe.'

If her testimony is not as spontaneous as this, remind her of the way she described her pain in the initial interview and show her a graphic depiction of her intensity levels (*Figure 12.3*). Explain the graph to her and work out, together, how it would have looked at the outset and compare that to the present graph. It could then become obvious that her condition has improved in an important aspect and she now needs less pain tablets.

Response to analgesics (R)

Correspondingly, the patient's analgesic response could have improved. One simple analgesic may now be as effective as were two compound analgesics initially.

Triggers

When one of the triggers is noticed to be less potent or impotent, the signs are good even if nothing else seems to have improved. For example, no premenstrual headache or no headache response to a stressful situation which previously would have precipitated or aggravated the headache. She should be reminded of the triggers she identified at her first interview and asked to compare her headache response to them now.

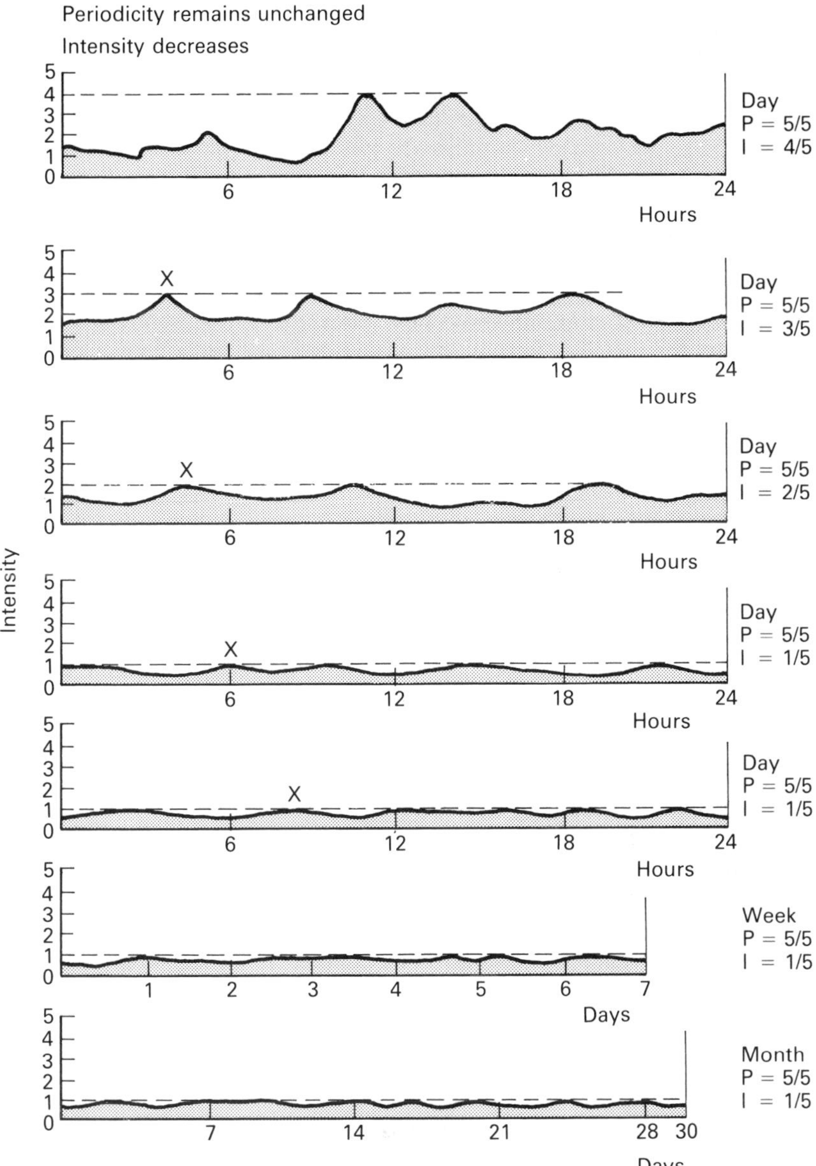

Figure 12.3 Assessment of pain: X indicates a treatment session

Associated symptoms

Nausea, dizziness, visual disturbances, etc. which may have been recorded initially as common concomitants of the headache may now be present less often or absent because these symptoms were usually present only when the pain was severe.

Because improvement can be detected in many small ways, and in difficult-to-assess cases one is dependent on these small indicators, it is especially important that as much information as possible is extracted. It should be elicited and recorded during the first visit so that it is available for detailed reassessment later. In particular when the periodicity factor is found to be erratic, care must be taken to record as many other potential reassessment details as possible for future use. Failure to do so will greatly diminish the possibility of success. The patient should be taught to assist with the monitoring of her headache by noticing and reporting small changes in the known pattern of her symptoms.

Physical signs

Re-evaluate the objective examination of the intervertebral joint source in greater depth. Has anything relevant been missed? Do a minutely exploring palpation of accessory movement of all possible joint sources from different approaches, different points of contact and aiming the pressures in other directions. Reassess also the physiological movements going into combination movements (Edwards, 1986) and palpate accessory intervertebral movements in different physiological positions.

Modify technique

Modify treatment techniques according to the new objective findings and increase the strength of application and duration of the technique. Make use of sustained stretching or distracting techniques.

Alternative mobilization techniques to try

Although most headaches respond well to a few simple techniques, it is necessary for those who offer to treat headaches to know a great many approaches to the offending joints and their restricted movement. It is necessary to be innovative and experimental in order to be successful with these reluctant cases. I have found the following techniques to be of use:

1. Transverse pressures on C1 in many directions and points of thumb contact.
2. Central postero-anterior pressure on C1 to C7.
3. C1 central postero-anterior pressure in a cephalad direction, digging underneath the base of the skull.
4. C1 unilateral postero-anterior pressure.
5. O/C1 manually applied distraction or compression.
6. O/C1 rotation.
7. O/C1 lateral flexion.

C2 to C6. All the above techniques can be tried, remembering that transverse pressures at these levels can be applied against the spinous process as well as against the articular pillar. In addition, postero-anterior pressures could be directed caudad as well as cephalad and unilateral postero-anterior pressures can be directed medially as well as in many other directions, also changing minutely the point of thumb contact.

C7. Pay particular attention to C7 as often, if its joints are tender to pressure, the headache will not clear until this joint has been dealt with. When carrying out unilateral postero-anterior pressures at C7 the pressure may be applied through the overlying muscle mass or, often more effectively, by hooking the thumbs underneath the muscle onto the posterior surface of the transverse process and moving it from there.

All the cervical facet joints may be moved in an anteroposterior direction and this technique applied to C1 and C2 is extremely useful. When applying anteroposterior pressures on the apophyseal joints of C1 and C2 one should place the thumbs anterior to the tendon of origin of the sternocleidomastoid, and for the lower cervical levels they should be posterior to it.

All tender thoracic and lumbar levels should be palpated for and treated until joint signs are cleared. Central postero-anterior and unilateral postero-anterior and transverse pressures should be tried, again in all directions and points of thumb contact.

Palpate and treat tender sacral and coccygeal joints too. Do not stop treatment until all vertebral signs are clear, by which time the headache should have cleared up.

Although pain cannot be anatomically referred from these levels to the head and the headache arises in a painful condition of the upper cervical spine, it is sometimes necessary to clear these lower joints before the headache will ultimately abate. One can only speculate on this clinical finding. It could be that painful lower levels cause protective spasm in the paravertebral muscles. As these muscles overlie all the vertebral joints the maintained contraction could reactivate the upper cervical symptoms. This may not be an acceptable explanation but it is clinically useful to know that some stubborn headaches clear up only after all the stiff or painful spinal joints have been mobilized.

Mobilize in particular O/C1/C2 in every possible direction. The following technique is especially useful in locating a covert headache-producing articulation.

Postero-anterior pressures along the base of the skull onto the arch of the atlas with progressive rotation of the head (O/C1)

This is not a technique described elsewhere but the reader will find it invaluable in locating the exact occipito-atlantal accessory movement in which a painful restriction of range is causing the headache.

The patient lies prone with her head extending about 5 cm over the end of the couch. Her hands rest over the end of the couch on either side of her head. She is asked to flex her neck strongly, tucking her chin well in and resting her forehead on the couch. The therapist stands at the patient's head, facing her feet. He places his right thigh against the crown of her head and asks her to accept the support offered and so relax her neck muscles and ligaments (*see Figure 12.4*). The therapist, using his thumbs, palpates the spinous process of C2 and then slides his thumbs down the superior surface onto the tubercle of the atlas. A straight postero-anterior pressure is exerted through the tough resistance of the

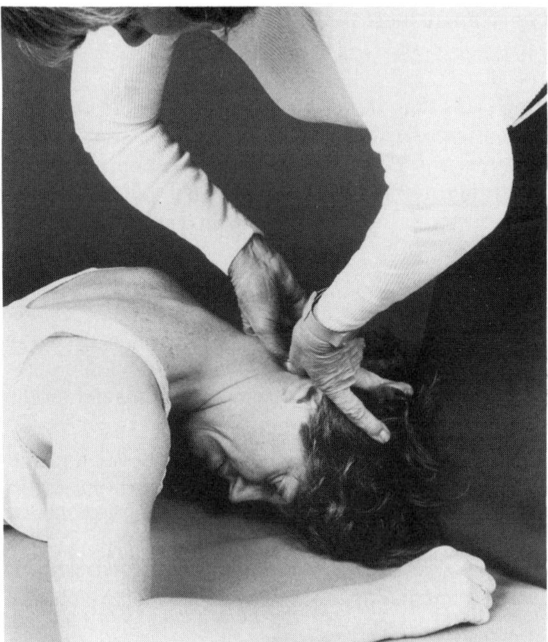

Figure 12.4 Unilateral postero-anterior pressures, moving progressively laterally while rotating the patient's head progressively more to the right. Pressures at each point are directed towards the head. The patient's head on the neck is supported in a strongly flexed position

ligamentum nuchae until the tubercle can be felt to move. This pressure should be exerted straight downwards and then digging under the skull in a cephalad direction. A sharp pain response is sought, which will identify the lesion.

If these pressures are sore but do not elicit a sharp response, move the thumbs about 0.5 cm to the right along the nuchal line, at the same time asking the patient to turn her head very slightly to the right while maintaining the chin-in position. Apply the postero-anterior and postero-anterior cephalad pressures in the way described above. Work along the base of the skull in this manner until full rotation is reached, ending thus with a transverse pressure towards the left on the tip of the transverse process of C1. No unresponsive headache should be discharged before the possibilities of positive signs have been examined in this way.

Use transverse pressures on the transverse process of C1 directed in every possible direction, also varying the point of thumb contact. Direct pressure towards the ipsilateral eye, the contralateral eye, the nose, the ipsilateral and the contralateral ear, the mouth, the chin, posteriorly towards the tubercle of the atlas and downwards towards the feet. Some or all of these may be tender to Grades I or II, but one of them may be markedly more sensitive and cause the patient to flinch or cry out. This then would indicate the therapeutic technique. The patient's ipsilateral eye should be constantly observed as the eye response is a good indicator of the intensity of pain experienced with each pressure. One could disregard the conventional grade gauge and apply, at each point, a pressure which records a minimal eye response, thus judging the most sensitive point to be that where the least pressure, sometimes even mere skin contact, causes it. The strength of pressure which causes minimal eye response should be used therapeutically.

All treatment pressures should be applied up to Grade IV +++ before being discarded. When treating these tender joints with, say, 20 Grade IV pressures, tell the patient what you mean to do and how many pressures you intend to carry out. Tell her that you will break the 20 pressures up into volleys of three or four each. This makes it easier for her to tolerate such painful treatment and is equally effective for treatment purposes.

When varying the directions of pressures it is interesting to note that in some situations a Grade IV pressure in a certain direction is quite comfortable whereas the most minute shift of contact or direction could elicit a sharp pain response.

These variations should also be applied from C2 to C7. Central postero-anterior pressures at C2 should be directed caudad, cephalad and also cephalad with a lateral inclination to the left and to the right. All cervical unilateral pressures should be tried in a medial direction, close to the spine and at the furthest limits of the transverse process and at every point in between.

C7 may be advantageously mobilized in a direction approaching the quadrant position for the lower cervical spine as follows.

C6 to T3 diagonal movement towards the right (in prone) Grades I to IV

The patient lies prone with her head fully rotated to the right, her right hand resting in front of her face and her right elbow moved further to the left so that her right shoulder drops into a relaxed position. Her left arm lies by her left side. The therapist stands behind her. He places the tip of his left thumb against the left lateral aspect of the spinous process of the vertebra below the joint to be manipulated, maintaining a straight line from the tip of his thumb to his elbow. He leans across the patient and places the heel of his right hand in contact with the inferior border of the patient's maxillary arch, maintaining the wrist in some degree of extension (*see Figure 12.5*). With his two forearms moving parallel and opposite to one another, he moves that level of the patient's spine into the range available in that position – this will be a combination of extension, right rotation and left side flexion. This technique is described by Stoddard (1969) and used as a Grade V thrust, but is also usefully employed in the grades of mobilization, Grades I to IV.

Thoracic techniques should be varied too. Grade V technique should be used in stubborn cases attempting to clear thoracic signs, particularly T4.

Lumbosacral, sacro-iliac and coccygeal articulations should be mobilized by means of direct pressures according to the most painful site and direction as established by palpation. I remember a patient, a young woman, with headache as the dominant symptom but also other minor vertebral symptoms for which she would not have sought treatment had they presented without the headache. Mobilization of the upper cervical spine abated the headache at each treatment session but it kept recurring. As I extended the treatment lower down the spine the remission of headache lengthened but the headaches did not altogether abate until I had cleared all the vertebral signs as far down as, and including, the coccyx.

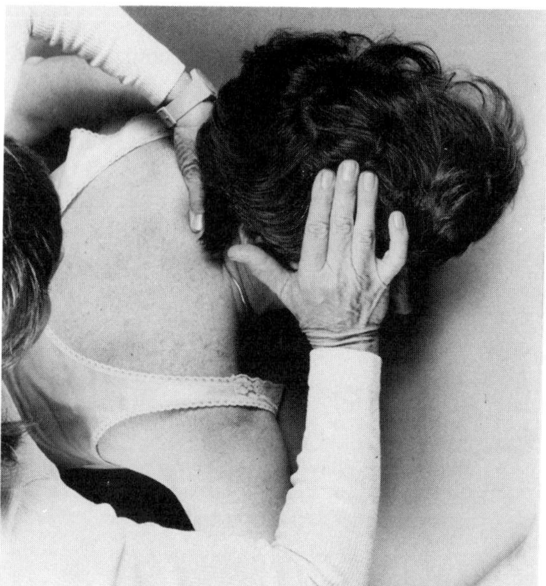

Figure 12.5 C6 to T3 diagonal movement towards the right (in prone) Grades I to IV

In using any of the techniques suggested in the foregoing it is best to start the palpation using Grade I pressures or movement and advance fairly rapidly to Grade IV and IV+ if no pain response is forthcoming. Use the treatment technique according to the tolerance of the joint. If it should become necessary to go to a Grade V during the course of treatment, which in stubborn cases it often is, remember first to check for contraindications to manipulation (*see* Chapter 15).

Palpation

Palpate and treat tender suboccipital thickenings with a modality of choice, for example deep transverse frictions according to Cyriax (1973). Palpate for and treat cervical muscle spasm and fibrous thickening at any level.

Traction

Traction does not help all headaches and sometimes makes them worse, but when dealing with a stubborn headache which does not respond to mobilization or manipulation it should be tried as in some cases it is the only treatment that is effective.

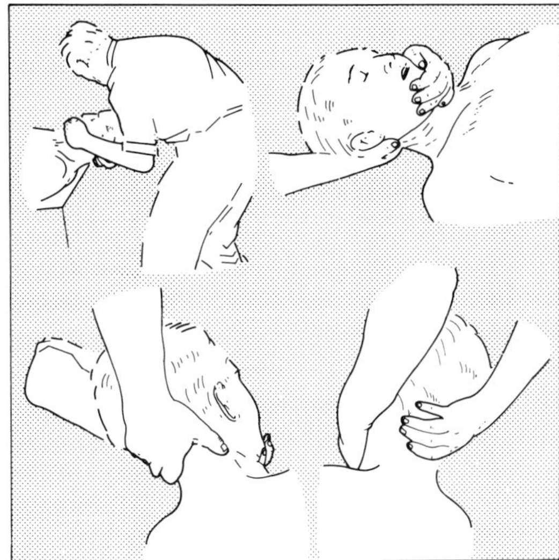

Figure 12.6 Longitudinal movement (←•→)

If the headache is currently present it is worthwhile carrying out the following test in order to establish whether traction is likely to be useful:

The patient lies supine with the upper cervical spine in a neutral position between flexion and extension and also between left and right side flexion and left and right rotation. The therapist grasps her head, placing one hand under her chin and the other under her occiput. He hugs the head and, using his body weight, exerts a longitudinal pull, starting with a small or moderate force (*see* Figure 12.6). Whilst maintaining the pull he asks the patient to report any change in the headache, for example does it:

Go away?
Become less severe?
Remain unaltered?
Become worse?

If it lessens or abates while the traction is applied, commence a regimen of traction as described by Maitland (*Vertebral Manipulation*, 5th edn., Chapter 9): to the upper cervical spine using the least poundage found to be effective.

Other physiotherapy modalities

Use any other physiotherapy modality such as heat, massage, ice, ultrasound, interferential current, transcutaneous electrical nerve stimulation, shortwave diathermy – all in conjunction with mobilization or manipulation.

Manipulation

Therapists who are expert at manipulating, whether as taught by Maitland or any other manipulator, could use the more forceful technique of Grade V manipulation on the upper cervical spine or at any level where stiffness is found, but only when gentler mobilization potential has been exhausted, and also only in the absence of contraindications.

Fortunately the cases which do not respond significantly are relatively few, but it does not comfort the unfortunate ones to know how successful we are with most cases like theirs. Nor does it comfort the therapist and we spend many sleepless nights wondering what we are doing wrong and what our next move should be. But if nothing avails, we must in turn abandon them too. No purpose is served by continuing useless treatment when there is not even temporary relief. Do not be discouraged but remind yourself of those whose lives you have improved by relieving them of the burden of pain.

Re-examine in terms of disorders of other musculoskeletal systems

Although the most common source of the non-vascular chronic headache is to be found in the joints of the upper cervical spine, other structures may be partly or fully responsible. This book describes in detail the author's approach and method of treatment of intervertebral joint disorders which refer pain into the head. Examination and treatment of such other musculoskeletal structures are well documented in other works: brief reference will be made to these where there is specific relevance to headache.

Temporomandibular joint

Test and incorporate suitable treatment (*see* Chapters 8 and 10 and Trott, 1986). When the head pain encroaches on the terrain of the lower two divisions of the trigeminal nerve, examine and treat, by mobilization, positive findings in the temporomandibular joint (TMJ) but take great care not to overtreat initially because the TMJ condition is often very irritable. (Trott and Goss, 1978; Rocabado, 1985; Selby, 1985; Helland, 1986; Trott, 1986)

Posture and muscular imbalance

Postural imbalance or 'poor posture' is seldom the primary cause of a severe pain syndrome like chronic headache. All who exhibit poor posture do not suffer headache or even backache. But it can play an important role in the production of symptoms and inhibit or diminish a favourable outcome of treatment by mobilization. In those cases which do not respond to mobilization alone the posture must be examined and its role in the condition evaluated.

Janda (1987) describes a situation where certain muscles become short and their antagonists long. When this is operative in the proximal part of the body there is tightness of the levator scapulae, upper trapezius and pectorals and weakness of the lower stabilizers of the scapulae and the deep neck flexors. The postural appearance is that of round shoulders, exaggerated low cervical forward flexion and craniovertebral extension – the 'chin-poke' posture. He calls this the 'proximal or shoulder crossed syndrome' and it has direct bearing on the condition of cervical headache.

This posture results in greatly increased pressure on the joints and other structures of the upper cervical spine, which is the main source of the cervical headache condition. This pressure is threefold, from:

1. Compression of the posterior aspect of the craniovertebral joint which occurs in upper cervical extension.
2. Tight, thickened and shortened muscles overlying the craniovertebral joints.
3. The weight of the skull and its contents which come to rest on the craniovertebral joints.

Because these joints are exceptionally sensitive to even slight pressure increase, this situation aggravates the headache and, if not corrected, will reactivate the syndrome even if it has responded well to initial treatment.

The posture should be demonstrated to the patient and corrective action taken. If the patient is asked to place her two index fingers along the base of her skull and then to allow her neck to slump forward into the chin-poke posture she will feel the weight of the skull come to rest on the craniovertebral joints which she will by this time have come to recognize as the source of her headache. She is then asked to retract the chin, lengthening the back of her neck and she will feel the cranium lifting off the pain source. This is a quick way to make her aware of the effect of the posture she adopts for so many hours a day at her desk or computer.

Exercises should be taught which will strengthen the deep neck flexors and shoulder retractors, thus lengthening the craniovertebral muscles and the patient should be motivated to carry them out. Furthermore, because the proximal crossover syndrome is often part of a general imbalance involving the whole body, the total posture must be evaluated for defect and corrected.

Passive mobilization of the shortened muscles

The patient lies supine. The therapist stands behind her head and encircles the patient's atlas with his left thumb and index finger, resting the dorsum of his hand on the couch. His right hand cradles the base of the skull in his palm, fingers and thumb. He completes this grasp by giving support to the head, with the anteromedial aspect of his right glenohumeral joint immediately below the clavicle.

Method

While holding the atlas quite still with his left hand grasp, the skull is lifted cephalad and anteriorly using the right hand to obtain the longitudinal movement and the right shoulder to tip the patient's head forward. This may be used as an oscillating technique or a maintained stretch. This technique is also used as a neuromeningeal stretch but very gently to avoid exacerbation of an irritable neural condition (*see* also Chapter 14).

Myofascial disorder

This is a painful condition of the skeletal muscles characterized by the presence of one or more discrete hyperaesthetic areas called trigger points, located within muscles or tendons; when stimulated by pressure, these trigger points produce pain in the area of the patient's symptoms (Dox et al., 1983; Barnes, 1990; Pullen, 1992a,b).

A chronic headache is sometimes caused, but more often augmented, by the myofascial condition. A great number of spinal muscles arise from or insert into the base of the occipital bone and these are susceptible to the development of myofascial pain and trigger points which refer pain into the head. These include trapezius, semispinalis capitis, superior oblique, rectus capitis posterior major and minor, occipitalis, sternomastoid, splenius capitis, longissimus capitis, digastric and rectus capitis lateralis. Deep palpation, exploring along and, as far as is possible, under the base of the skull will reveal the tendinous 'twitch response' points (Travell and Simons, 1983). These are effectively treated by the ischaemic pressure technique described by Travell, where the trigger point is isolated within the tendon with the muscles in a stretched position. The patient's feedback should be sought in the identification of the trigger point which reproduces the headache. Thumb pressure is maintained and the patient asked to say when the pain begins to recede from the head area, then when the local pain diminishes and then when the pain has gone and she is only aware of the pressure.

Many of the trigger points will be situated very deeply and are not easily accessible. One way to reach them is to position the patient as is described earlier in this chapter for the technique headed: 'Postero-anterior pressures along the base of the skull onto the arch of the atlas with progressive rotation of the head'. This is a mobilizing technique but instead of mobilizing in this position a deep palpation is carried out seeking to explore under the rim of the skull in order to identify and compress trigger points.

Trigger points should also be sought in the bellies of any of these muscles, particularly in the trapezius, splenius capitis, supra- and infrahyoid muscles, all of which may be a source of cranial, cervical and facial pain. Splenius capitis trigger points are often responsible for a complaint of dizziness and ischaemic pressures as described are very effective.

Tension in myofascial tissue in these and more distant muscles may be explored and treated with the deep release (cross-hand) or other techniques described by Barnes (1990). The occipital condyle and cervical release techniques are effective in releasing suboccipital tension.

Dural or extrasegmental pain

Cyriax (1973) believes that 'trigger points', 'myalgic spots' and 'fibrositis' are not primary lesions but secondary phenomena to pressure on the dura mater, leading to extrasegmental pain and tenderness and suggests that massage and injections applied to these spots are inappropriate and that treatment should be directed to the joint source. But in cases where mobilization alone has been ineffective, the author has found trigger point therapy to be effective.

Adverse mechanical tension

The author has more recently become aware of the significance of the involvement of the central nervous system as a complication of some cervical articular headaches. Since attending a course given by Gwendolen Jull, based on the research of, inter alia, Janda, Butler and Elvey, the author has been assessing and treating tension and tethering of the neural tissue and also postural muscle imbalance. This has added a further dimension to the prognosis of those cases who respond poorly to the treatment of the joints alone. It is important to assess, in cases which respond poorly, signs of adverse mechanical tension (AMT) in nervous tissue (Butler, 1987) and also muscle imbalance, altered movement patterns and trigger points referring pain (Janda, 1987).

This book sets out to describe the examination and treatment by joint mobilization of the chronic headache which arises in the cervical spine; the scope does not allow for adequate information on examination and treatment of AMT. Thorough knowledge and experience in such testing and treatment is necessary for the therapist who attempts the treatment of chronic headache by this route. Rather than supply abbreviated information, which could encourage superficial examination and assessment the author refers the reader to Breig (1977). Breig examines the effects of the pathological forces that deform the soft tissues in the spinal canal. New concepts of basic biomechanics and of neuropathology are outlined. Although this book is aimed at neurosurgeons the basic principles of this research should be understood by therapists who seek to treat pain conditions arising from neural tissue tension. The cranial and cervical dura are pain sensitive and can be a source of headache and especially so if the patient has had previous invasive surgery. One of the most severe cases of chronic headache in my experience was a post-whiplash case who had had four surgical procedures carried out on the cervical spine and two manipulations under general anaesthetic. All tension tests were positive at the beginning of range. All attempts at mobilizing the neural tissue gave rise to extreme exacerbation of her headache.

Neural tissue tension is a component in a limited number of cases of chronic headache and its presence would be suggested by a positive response to tests which examine the free movement of the spinal cord and its investments within the intervertebral canal. These are:

Passive head/neck flexion
Straight leg raise (SLR)
Prone knee bend
Upper limb tension test 1 (ULTT) (Elvey, 1985, 1986)
Upper limb tension test 2
Slump (Maitland, 1986)
Slump test in long sitting.

Any of these tests is positive if the test reproduces the patient's headache and further examination and treatment should be guided by the approaches set out by Elvey (1986) and Butler (1987, 1991). It should be assumed that it is an irritable condition, until proved otherwise.

One simple technique which I use in some cases which resist treatment by mobilization and which is also described by Butler (1991) is palpation of nerves. It would be appropriate, for headache, to palpate the greater occipital nerve and, if tight or tender and if it refers pain, to massage or friction the nerve and surrounding connective tissue, or to apply oscillating pressures or static ischaemic pressure as to a trigger point. The same could be done with the trigeminal nerve and its branches.

It should be born in mind that mobilization of vertebral joints forms part of the treatment regime for neural tissue tightness and that some of the success achieved by mobilization could, in cases with AMT involvement, be due partly to the incidental mobilization of neural tissue.

Re-examination by specialists in other medical fields

Most of these cases will have been medically examined and treated before reaching the therapist. It would be worthwhile to discuss the results of previous tests at this stage or to request further tests, for example a full medical and neurological examination and a routine laboratory profile. Diagnostic studies such as computerized tomography or magnetic resonance imaging will be used selectively. The patient then reverts to the care of the medical doctors, unless the indications are that physical therapy should be continued or modified to support the medical or surgical treatment ensuing from tests.

Vascular, inflammatory, neurological or intracranial sources or components are sought which might be causing or contributing to the poor response (Mondell, 1991).

Non-responders

These cases should be referred to experts in the following fields: pain clinics; neurology; neurosurgery; psychiatry; biofeedback; acupuncture; hypnosis.

References

Barnes, J., ed. (1990) *Myofascial Release. A Comprehensive Evaluatory and Treatment Approach.* MFR Seminary, New York

Breig, A., ed. (1977) *Adverse Mechanical Tension in the Central Nervous System*, pp. 115, 117, 140. John Wiley and Sons, New York

Butler, D. (1991) *Mobilisation of the nervous system.* Churchill Livingstone, London

Butler, D. S. (1987) A concept and treatment of adverse mechanical tension in the nervous system – application to repetition strain injury. In *Proceedings of the 5th Biennial Conference of the Australian Manipulative Therapists Association.* pp. 247–267

Cyriax, J., ed. (1973) Treatment by manipulation, massage and injection. In *Textbook of Orthopaedic Medicine*, Vol. 2, 8th edn., pp. 18–22. Baillière and Tindall, London

Dox, I., Melloni, B. J. and Eisner, G. M. (1983) *Melloni's Illustrated Medical Dictionary*, Williams and Wilkens, Baltimore

Edeling, J. (1974) Migraine and other chronic headaches. *South African Journal of Physiotherapy*, **36**, 13–17

Edeling, J. (1986) The abandoned headache syndrome. In Grieve, G. P., ed., *Modern Manual Therapy*. Churchill Livingstone, Edinburgh

Edwards, B. C. (1986) Examination of the high cervical spine (occiput-C2) using combined movements. In Greive, G. P., ed, *Modern Manual Therapy*, Churchill Livingstone, Edinburgh

Elvey, R. L. (1985) Brachial Plexus Tension Tests and the Pathoanatomical origin of Arm Pain. In *Aspects of Manipulative Therapy* 2nd ed. (Ed. E. F. Glasgow, L. T. Twomey *et al*) Churchill Livingstone

Elvey, R. L. (1986) Treatment of arm pain associated with abnormal brachial plexus tension. *Australian Journal of Physiotherapy*, **32**, 225–230

Helland, M. M. (1986) Anatomy and function of the temporomandibular joint. In Grieve, G. P. ed. *Modern Manual Therapy of the Vertebral Column*, Churchill Livingstone, Edinburgh

Janda, V. (1987) Muscles and cervicogenic pain syndromes in physical therapy of the cervical and thoracic Spine. In Grant, R., ed., *Clinics in Physical Therapy*, Vol. 17. Longman, London

Maitland, G. D., ed. (1986) *Vertebral Manipulation*, 5th edn. Butterworth, London

Melloni, B. J. and Eisner, G. M., eds (1979) *Melloni's Medical Dictionary*. Williams and Wilkins, Baltimore

Mondell, B. E. (1991) Evaluation of the patient presenting with headache. *Medical Clinics North America*, **75**, (3) 521–524

Pullen, S. I. (1992a) 1. Myofascial pain: a review. *South African Journal of Physiotherapy* **48**, 23–25

Pullen, S. I. (1992b) 2. Myofascial pain: a review. Part two: trigger points. *South African Journal of Physiotherapy*, **48**, 37–39

Rocabado, M., ed. (1985) *Arthrokinematics of the Temporomandibular Joint in Clinical Management of Head, Neck and TMJ Pain and Dysfunction*. W. B. Saunders, London

Selby, A. (1985) Physiotherapy in the management of temporomandibular disorders. *Australian Dental Journal*, **30**, (4) 273–280

Stoddard, A. (1969) *Manual of Osteopathic Practice*, Hutchison Medical Publications, London.

Travell, J. G. and Simons, M. D., eds. (1983) *Myofascial Pain and Dysfunction. The Trigger Point Manual*. Williams and Wilkins, Baltimore

Trott, P. H. (1986) Examination of the temporomandibular joint. In Grieve, G. P., ed., *Modern Manual Therapy*. Churchill Livingstone, Edinburgh

Trott, P. H. and Goss, A. N. (1978) Physiotherapy in diagnosis and treatment of the myofascial pain dysfunction syndrome. *International Journal of Oral Surgery* **7**, 360–365

Further reading

Bogduk, N. (1986) The cervical causes of headache and dizziness. In Grieve, G. P., ed., *Modern Manual Therapy of the Vertebral Column*. Churchill Livingstone, Edinburgh

Elvey, R. L. (1983) Treatment of conditions accompanied by signs of abnormal brachial plexus tension. In *Proceedings Neck and Shoulder Symposium*, MTAA, Brisbane

13

Post-discharge management

Let us assume that the patient has responded to treatment and the time has come to stop. It would be most unwise to discharge the patient finally because at this stage there is no way of knowing which of the following situations will prevail. The possibilities are:

1. *Maximum response*. The symptoms do not recur and the patient will require no more treatment in the future. The therapist, once he has gained experience in this form of treatment, can expect over 70% of chronic headache cases to respond to this extent.
2. *Good response*. In this group the syndrome will recur after a long period, even a few years. Often it will recur as a result of adverse circumstances which could involve an injury or excessive emotional or physical stress. The same treatment which caused the initial syndrome to abate could be expected to have the same effect once more.
3. *Fair response*. The headache, although it appears initially to have abated, still occurs but with a reduced periodicity pattern. Often it is also less severe when it does occur and responds better to simple analgesics and so the patient is able to accept it. Whereas a patient with a headache of, say, P = 4/5 or 5/5, I = 4/5 and R = 4/5 (TPP = 12 + /15) will be unable to conduct a normal lifestyle, she would be able to cope with an I = 3/5 headache once a week which abates when she takes two Disprins. This would be portrayed in a pain pattern of: P = 2/5, I = 3/5 and R = 1/5 (TPP = 6/15).

   If this pattern begins to build up again and to impinge more on her lifestyle, she should return for treatment until the TPP is again reduced to a satisfactory level. In some cases the recurrences will become less and less frequent with this management but others might need to be treated permanently on this basis. The desirability of permanent treatment must be weighed against the amount of analgesic which would otherwise be required and the harm that this could cause.
4. *Poor response*. Some cases of headaches, although they respond readily to each treatment, have a very poor carry-over period. It is debatable whether one is justified in treating them as often as they recur. If no other treatment has afforded any relief at all and regular and permanent treatment will enable the patient to reduce her drug intake significantly it would seem right to do so, provided that the patient agrees that it is worth her while. One should probably cope with the mild or moderate headaches even if they occur frequently but would seek help for a very severe bout. I think it is important for the patient to know that the therapist will be available to her at any time when she calls for help, simply because, by the time that she decides to call, she will be desperate and it would be callous to offer her an appointment on the following

day. It is important to be available for such cases because when the headache is so bad no relief can be obtained from analgesics or rest. The therapist would dispose of the only treatment other than morphine that could give relief to a patient who is feeling suicidal.

5. *No response*. Some cases, and fortunately they are few, do not respond in any way to any form of treatment applied to the neck. Because they have also failed to respond to the treatment of many other specialists there seems to be nothing one can do for them. Nevertheless they cause us sleepless nights before we finally tell them, as we must, that we are unable to help and that they must return to their referring doctor. There is no point in continuing treatment once you have exhausted all your strategies and there has been no response at all.

After discharge the patients of group 1 will not return for treatment of headache. If you wish to know whether they have remained subsymptomatic you would have to contact them for follow-up purposes. This is a very worthwhile exercise and the therapist gets to know the order of his results. For these patients it would not have mattered whether the therapist had told them or not to report recurrences, and if one knew at that time who they were going to be it would be unnecessary to do so. But because there is no way of knowing at the time of discharge into which group they will fall, it is very necessary to tell each patient that she may have recurrences and that if she does she should report back for more of the same treatment. Tell her also that there is no limit to the number of times that this treatment may be safely repeated because it is so gentle and does not involve anaesthetics or drugs.

At the commencement of treatment the patient should not have been led to expect a miraculous cure. One should have told her that she has a certain lesion which has been causing her headache and that arthritis cannot be cured but that you expect to be able to render the condition less painful or quite pain-free; and that a recurrence after successful treatment is not unusual and does not mean that the treatment has failed but only that it requires more of the same. Tell her that in the case of a severe recurrence you would be available to see her at short notice. This is very reassuring for the patient who turns out to be a fair or a poor responder and she no longer feels abandoned nor does she live in fear of recurrence of a condition which had become more than she could bear. She should not be made to feel a nuisance if she should need frequent booster treatments. She will feel self-conscious about bothering the therapist at inconvenient times and I find that these patients do not abuse the facility. They tend to hold back over weekends or at night unless they really are unable to cope. It is no hardship for a practitioner to hold himself available for certain emergencies and those who offer to treat chronic headache should cater for the possibility of occasional inconvenience.

At discharge it is not wise to tell the patient to avoid the circumstances which had previously resulted in an exacerbation of headache. It is better to attempt to improve the joint condition to such an extent that it is no longer as sensitive to the precipitating factors, which is the condition the joint had been in for many years before the escalation of the syndrome in spite of the presence of the lesion. By the time she is ready for discharge this fact should be evident, for example, she could have reported that an emotional upset of the sort that would have triggered a headache before commencement of treatment no longer had this effect. Alternatively, she might report the absence of her usual premenstrual headache. These observations are reliable indications that the lesion is less irritable and that the joint is behaving more like a normal joint. It might, however, still respond with headache when subjected to a very strong precipitant, e.g. a major emotional crisis such as divorce or bereavement, excessive pressure of work or anxiety, but not by the normal everyday stresses present in everyone's life.

A patient who repeatedly returns with recurrence of symptoms related to minor stress would be a person whose stress tolerance is low and who responds with excessive muscular reaction to even trifling levels of stress. In such cases it is beneficial to make the patient aware of the cervical muscle contraction operative in the presence of stress and to teach her to counter it with a voluntary decontraction when it occurs. Sometimes this is insufficient to reduce the adverse effects of stress but in very tense subjects it would be necessary to teach them how to relax and continue to do so until they are able to reduce their stress response.

Some patients in groups 3 and 4 above have a headache which consistently abates with the application of a very simple technique. It is sometimes useful to teach the patient or a member of her family how to carry out this technique and so make her self-sufficient in coping with recurrences. One should especially try to do this for people who might have come a long distance for treatment and who are returning home.

In any sample of headache cases there will be a variable individual response which the therapist will only be able to assess fully some time after discharge and so it becomes very important for the patient to report recurrences. In this way she will derive the benefit of the maximum possible control of the syndrome which need not get out of hand again as it had been at the time when she first presented for treatment.

The importance of post-discharge management

If the patient does not understand the various ways in which her syndrome can behave after discharge, she might not return to avail herself of that which is possibly the only treatment which will ever give significant and reliable relief. Remember:

- She has seen many doctors and specialists and has submitted to many expensive tests and treatments to no avail.

- She is aware of the fact that eminent medical specialists do not seem to know what is causing her headaches and some have suggested that she is neurotic and in some way causing her own headache.

- She has been to fringe and lay practitioners and has had certain treatments which have helped for a period of weeks or months, e.g. chiropractors, acupuncturists and reflexologists. Surgery might have given only a limited period of relief but the headaches came back.

So if you do not tell her what to expect and what to do if they should recur she is likely to sink back into her depressive state and suffer on alone, resorting to analgesic abuse. She could feel too embarrassed to admit of yet another failure, fearing that this may finally confirm her hypochondria.

Only recently I had a case which illustrates the need for post-discharge management. A distressed sounding woman telephoned me to ask for an urgent appointment. Her headache was driving her mad, she said, and she could not stand it any longer. I made time to see her and when she arrived she told me the following story:

> Five years before she had been treated by me for a severe headache syndrome. It had cleared up under that treatment and had remained clear for four years. Then she had a recurrence of headache together with some other disorder. The disorder, for which she sought medical help, cleared up but the headache remained. When she repeatedly returned to her doctor to report the persisting headache, which had not responded at all to his medication, he suggested that it was 'all in the mind'. This made her angry, she said, but because she had to be sure, she agreed to consult a psychiatrist. He tried to convince her that she suffered from a deep-seated depression but she disagreed. She was a contented woman and had no need to be depressed. She was happily married, had good children and enjoyed her job (her words). She was then sent to the hospital outpatient department for tests. She had blood tests, sonar scans, X-rays, a brain scan and was seen by many specialists. The outcome was inconclusive and treatment attempts ineffective. A year went by in her quest for diagnosis and help before she remembered that I had relieved her similar headache five years before. That was when she phoned me.

I took out her file of five years back and as the headache was comparable repeated the treatment given then. The headache subsided and after the treatment was minimal. The following day she said that it had gone away altogether later in the day and had not returned. I repeated that treatment and there has been no recurrence.

Perhaps I had not sufficiently impressed upon this woman the need for reporting recurrence or perhaps she wanted to be quite sure that there was nothing more sinister behind her headache, but whatever the case she suffered unnecessarily for a year.

14

Prophylactic measures and self help

Initially it is not necessary or wise to introduce advice or coping mechanisms. The treatment is passive and signs of treatment response are sought and assessed under the same circumstances as those under which the headache had been current or worsening. If then, as a result of treatment, the patient is able to live her normal daily life without headache she may be discharged. In most cases no more treatment or instruction will be necessary as the condition had responded to quite passive mobilization. Even if she exhibits a poor posture or appears, to the practitioner, to be a 'tense' person it is usually not necessary to train her in the prophylactic correction of these faults. If her headache is gone and no longer is a problem, she will not be motivated to carry out an exercise or relaxation regime and much time will be wasted in teaching her these. Headache sufferers will be pleased to be free of the disabling headache and eager to get on with their lives and will forget all about the headache. After all, everyone who is 'tense' does not experience headache and nor do all of those with poor posture. She should, however, be told to report recurrences and if the condition seems to be building up again to seek more of the treatment which gave her relief before.

If it is assessed, on the patient's first return, that the improvement had maintained for a significant period until the condition had been reactivated by some physically or emotionally traumatic experience, the practitioner should repeat the same technique and procedure as had been effective before and expect the same result. The patient should be discharged when the syndrome is once more under control and again told to report recurrences.

Therapeutic self help

If there had been a good response to a simple technique, the patient may be taught how to use it herself. A technique which is very often effective and which patients can usually manage is transverse pressure against the tip of the transverse process of C1 (*see* Chapter 10). The patient should be taught to perform it and told to try it when she feels a headache coming on. She should apply 10 pressures and reassess the pain before trying more. She may use this whenever necessary. Another technique is unilateral postero-anterior pressures on C2 or on the lateral arch of C1 (*see* Chapter 10). Provided the patient is shown to keep her thumb and wrist rigid so as to apply the strength from the elbow, the technique should be effective. A spouse may also be taught to perform these techniques.

For those who have shown incomplete or poor response during the treatment period and for those in whom the condition repeatedly recurs it becomes necessary for the therapist to seek out and address the perpetuating factors (*see* Chapter 12). The search for other pathology is undertaken either during the initial course of treatment in the case of poor responders or at a later stage when the patient, having been discharged after successful treatment, reports frequent recurrences. Suitable treatment modification is instituted then.

Many factors, though not the cause, contribute to the perpetuation of a chronic headache syndrome. These usually involve stress-induced muscle tension and/or the impact that certain postures and activities related to a particular lifestyle exert on the headache lesion. A specific home programme will need to be devised for each patient. It is necessary to enlist the patient's cooperation and this will largely depend on the level of understanding of her condition and also her motivation. This section deals with the teaching, by the therapist, of coping skills to patients who respond poorly to passive treatment. Physical therapists are well versed in the teaching of relevant home care programmes in the ongoing management of musculoskeletal conditions but, because headache is such a unique syndrome (*see* Chapter 3), it requires some modification of emphasis to the usual routine and what follows applies more specifically to headache.

The patient will, by this time, have been given an understanding by the therapist of her condition (Chapter 5). Her understanding now becomes even more relevant as she will be expected to take part in the management of her problems. She will show more interest at this stage and be more motivated, realizing that passive treatment alone has been inadequate. Whether or not the chronic cervicogenic headache had been explained to her before it is good to reinforce that which she already knows. It must be done in terms that a layman can easily understand and she should be able to repeat the explanation to her family. Most patients are able to understand the simplified explanations outlined in Chapter 5.

Because the most common headache trigger is *stress* it is likely to be the most potent perpetuating factor and if the patient does not learn to control stress, her headaches are likely to recur even after a successful course of treatment. The patient should understand how stress affects her headache (Chapter 5).

Although the most common factors which perpetuate headache are those already mentioned, many headache sufferers will have individual, personalized triggers. Refer back to the patient's original assessment notes to see what the patient had previously identified as *her* headache triggers and work on those.

Stress

Coping with stress-induced tension

Show the patient, on a model of the cervical spine with the base of the skull attached, where the headache source is (O–C1–C2). Remind her how tender these are and how sensitive to pressure – by palpating them. Let her feel the spino-occipital muscles which overlie these joints. Show her a picture of them from an anatomy book. Refer her to Chapter 5 and go through the explanation of "How stress affects your headache" with her.

It is important to become aware of the presence of the tension. Many people are quite unaware of the presence of even severe tension and are surprised when it is brought to their attention. Others are aware of the fact that they are tense but do not know what to do about it. Self help begins with teaching an awareness of the stress and the ensuing muscle tension.

Short-term or minor stress

Teach awareness of muscle tension in response to stressful irritations. Describe some typical stress-inducing incidences, for example:

An angry dog rushing at you
Hearing a burglar in the house
A near-miss motor prang
A dressing down from the boss
A child screaming
Unsatisfactory service
The car breaking down
Rushing about or too much to do
Working to a deadline
Working when tired
Being caught in a traffic snarl
Frustration for any reason.

The therapist allows the patient to feel the stress response by placing her (the patient's) hands softly over the trapezius area of the therapist while he produces the contraction to be felt here in response to one such incident. She should then be asked to imagine herself in a like situation, preferably one to which she can relate. She should mime the stress response a couple of times while feeling it on herself with her own hands. Then tell her to hold that contraction strongly for a little while to become thoroughly aware of it and then, taking a deep breath, to slowly allow the contraction to relax whilst releasing her breath. Suggest that she imagines the muscles to be 'butter melting in hot sun'.

Having become acquainted with the perception of a strong contraction, she is then allowed to feel, on the therapist, a less strong contraction and then a minimal contraction. This is necessary for perception training. It is easier to be aware of strong muscle tension than of milder or minimal tension. A strong muscle contraction soon lessens to become a lesser contraction which is sustained and it takes practice to be able to perceive a minimal contraction and to be able to relax that too. This is very important because it is the maintained minor tension over a long period which perpetuates the headache. She should be taught this and told to practise it as an exercise. The therapist should check her progress and reinforce the importance of this exercise at each visit.

What irritates one person does not necessarily irritate another. It is useful to go back to the original assessment of the particular patient's condition and to remind her of the stress factors which were inclined to trigger her headache or make it worse. Ask her whether she can add to this list. Teach her then, to become aware of similar situations as they arise and to notice the resulting tension response in

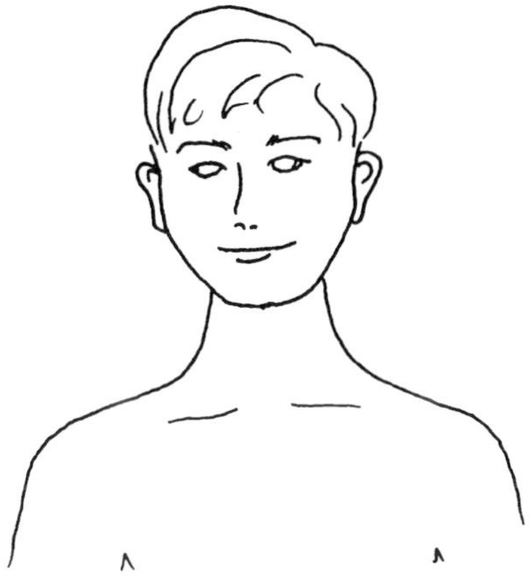

Figure 14.1 Muscles of neck and shoulder girdle relaxed

her neck. Having noticed it, to take in a long breath through her mouth and as she lets it out to let the tension melt away and then to deal with the crisis or the worry in a relaxed manner (*see Figure 14.1*).

Teach her also to be aware of situations during which it is common for anyone to maintain a tense neck and shoulder girdle (*see Figure 14.2*). Demonstrate that it is quite possible to drive in traffic with the shoulders relaxed instead of drawing them upwards towards the ears. The same applies to watching a thrilling movie, to studying or to writing an examination. Or to beating an egg or brushing one's teeth or scrubbing the floor. We tend also to hunch up in cold weather or walking in the rain. Or when we wait impatiently in a queue. Notice all the hunched shoulders round a conference table or among spectators of an exciting ball game. It is not necessary to avoid these situations, most of which form part of everyday life. But if she is able to recognize them and to defuse the muscle response she will have less headache. She should learn that these muscles are under her own control; that the muscles may be contracted *and* relaxed by her own volition. She might have been given muscle relaxant drugs in the past. Explain that those drugs relax *all* the body muscles. Show her that she is able to relax any voluntary group

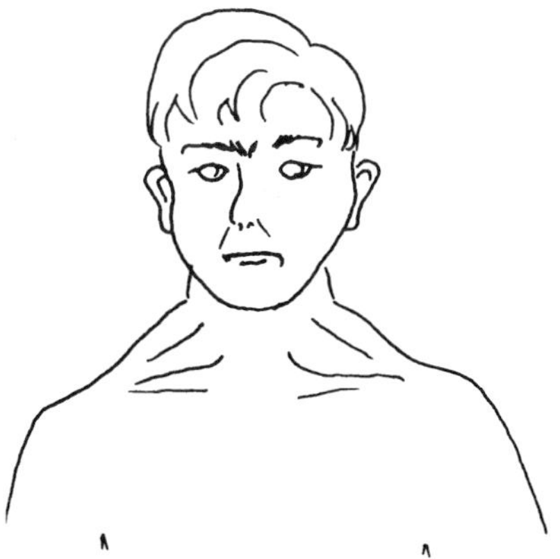

Figure 14.2 Muscle contraction in neck and shoulder girdle in stressful situation

of muscles selectively and that she will be able to help herself if she knows which muscles are aggravating her headache and is able to relax those and keep them relaxed. This is better than using a muscle relaxant drug in that she does not have to feel groggy because of the drug-induced relaxation.

The situations described above are those which form part of the fibre of daily living and the coping mechanisms described above will combat their ill effects.

Ongoing or chronic stress

Bereavement, shock, prolonged anxiety, insurmountable problems, unhappy work situations or marriage – these are stress forms which go beyond the minor irritations of daily living. A breadwinner who has been retrenched or an executive who is subjected to high levels of pressure might need more than the measures suggested above: they would benefit from a course of relaxation training and not all physical therapists are able to provide this. Such patients and also those who suffer stress associated with psychoses will require more specialized relaxation training.

Much can be achieved, however, if the therapist is able to modify the patient's attitudes. With patience and insight the patient may be encouraged to soften self-imposed standards. Some people drive themselves relentlessly, thus maintaining unnecessary levels of tension. Learning to recognize this and to become aware of the resultant tension and then being able to relax is more effective, and safer, than having to rely on drugs.

Posture

Understanding posture

Patients will have individual perceptions of what is a 'good' posture, which will reflect earlier conditioning by mothers, school teachers or army sergeants. They often give up in confusion and so should be taught by their therapist something of the biomechanics of posture and relate it to their particular postures and how these affect their symptoms.

Normal posture

Explain to the patient:

> 'The spine of an upright human has more curves than that of a four-footed creature such as a dog. These curves are an evolutionary adaptation to the vertical posture and the spinal structures have long since become adapted to the new alignment which has become the 'normal' human posture. Essentially the cervical spine curves forwards, the dorsal spine backwards and the lumbar spine forwards. Your therapist may show you a model of the spine, or drawings to illustrate these curves.

Slumping in a sitting position alters the cervical alignment into an extension of the upper and forward flexion of the lower cervical spine. This posture becomes operative in many static activities such as studying, writing, driving.'

Poor posture is often the result of muscle imbalance from various causes. Your therapist will analyse your posture and if there is muscle or other structural imbalance, will show you how to correct it or improve it with specific exercises.'

It is common for young girls who are very tall or who have large and heavy breasts to stoop. The round-shouldered posture adopted also adversely alters the neck posture and must be corrected. Poor posture can also be the long-term result of debilitating illness, depression or even personality traits such as those of submissiveness or timidity. In order to correct the posture these underlying causes need to be dealt with too.

The most common precipitant of the cervicogenic headache after stress, is the effect of incorrect and prolonged head-on-neck posture. The worst posture in relation to cervicogenic headache is undoubtedly the chin-poke posture.

Dealing with the chin poke

Observe the lateral view of the patient's posture and let her see it in a mirror or by the therapist demonstrating it or in a drawing (*Figure 14.3*). Draw her attention to and demonstrate the *forward head* position. Show the compensatory posterior rotation of the *head-on-neck*. Show her then that the head must be moved backward to be above and not in front of the shoulders and the chin tipped in so that the face is parallel to the wall. In this posture the head is balanced above the shoulders and the neck muscles are able to relax (*Figure 14.4*).

The patient must be made aware of a faulty posture and made to understand how the chin-poke posture affects her headache source, i.e. the craniovertebral structures. The following strategies are often helpful:

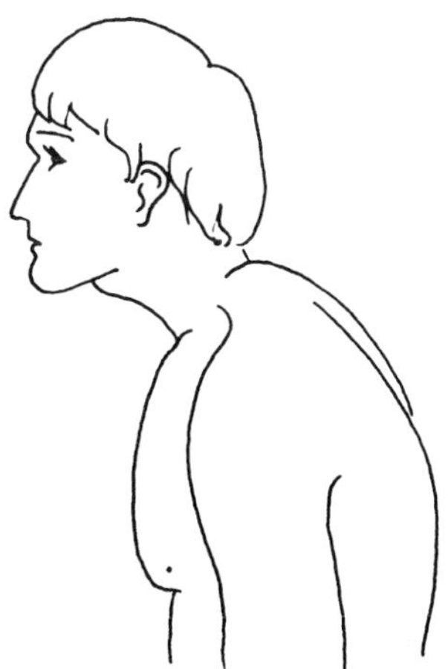

Figure 14.3 The chin-poke posture

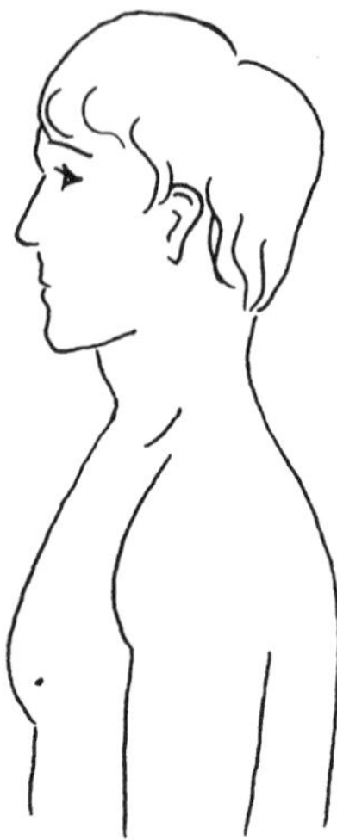

Figure 14.4 Correct head-on-neck posture with relaxed neck muscles

> Place the fingers softly over the craniovertebral area. Allow the chin to poke forward and feel how the weight of the skull comes to rest on the craniovertebral joints exerting pressure sufficient to trigger a headache when maintained. Feel also the shortening and thickening of the suboccipital structures which add to the pressure. Ask her then to reverse the posture, drawing the chin in and the head back and up. Feel the skull lift off the craniovertebral joints, relieving the pressure.

Explain also that if this is an habitual posture the craniovertebral muscles and other structures become shortened, lessening the ability to completely relieve the pressure. It will then become necessary to do, on a regular basis, certain exercises which tend to restore their normal length and to strengthen and shorten the short neck flexor muscles which had become lengthened and weakened. The following two exercises are effective:

> Lying supine, without a pillow, the patient draws the chin in strongly so as to make several double chins. Keeping the chin in she attempts to raise the head fractionally by tipping the crown of the head up without lifting the chin forward. This is a difficult exercise, especially for those with shortened suboccipital structures and needs to be practised under supervision until the patient masters it; then she should do it at home a few times every day.
>
> An easier exercise is done whilst lying prone. The head and shoulders are raised off the couch while the shoulders are held depressed and back, approximating the shoulder blades. The head is held back with the chin tucked in so that the head and neck is in line with the dorsal spine. This must be repeatedly practised, corrected and performed at home several times a day.

The patient should be encouraged to correct the chin poke constantly if it has become an habitual posture as shown in *Figure 14.4*. Fashion models are taught to imagine they are scraping the ceiling with the crown of their head when they walk. This is an easy and effective way of bringing the posture into good alignment.

Remedying adverse occupational postures

In order to maintain eye focus for static occupational pursuits the head must be fixed in a particular position for unnaturally long periods. Because these functions require concentration, the person is distracted and fails to alter the position when the neck puts out warnings that it is beginning to feel the strain which, if prolonged, will result in headache. By the time the headache develops it is too late.

The harmful effect of many occupational postures is compounded by concomitant stress, for example driving a car under adverse conditions. Driving is very often given as one of the precipitants of the patient's headache. In such cases the patient should be advised to address both components, by monitoring the muscle tension reaction as suggested above and by maintaining a correct neck posture. She should also move the neck often. Show her that the neck may be moved in all directions whilst not taking her eyes off the road. When driving long distances, frequent stops or changing drivers is essential.

Teach the patient the importance of being aware of posture during other static occupational activities. Suggest ways of arranging the work station to minimize adverse effects. Analyse each patient's activity and together work out modifications which will achieve a posture which does not strain the spine.

It is wise for her to introduce frequent breaks in her work, if only to look up and down and around, shrug and circle the shoulder girdle and then to continue only after she has made sure that the posture is correct and the shoulder girdle muscles relaxed. This takes seconds only and aborts hours of unnecessary pain. Some will need to devise a reminder, for example to break at the end of every page, or tie a red ribbon to a finger or even use an electronic timer which buzzes.

Lifting

Lifting and carrying heavy objects exerts strain on the shoulder/neck muscles which in turn results in overloading strain of cervical joints. The muscles which stabilize the shoulder girdle in order to enable the arms to handle weights attach to the transverse processes of the cervical vertebrae above and to the shoulder blade below. (The therapist should show an anatomical illustration of these muscles and it will be clear how lifting can have a bad effect on the headache source.)

The patient should avoid unnecessary lifting and carrying. Small children can be taught to climb onto one's lap instead of being lifted from the floor. The patient must be willing to admit that she has a condition which is aggravated by lifting any weight. Many people, especially men, are unwilling to admit to this weakness and cause themselves much resulting pain which could have been avoided. Shopping is often implicated in the worsening of cervical symptoms. It is better to make some contingency plan than to regularly suffer the consequences in a martyr-like fashion. The patient should do something to lessen the load on her neck. It is cumulative. The following tips may be useful:

Using a push basket instead of carrying
Getting someone who does not have a cervical problem to assist or do the shopping

Buying small quantities at a time
Some stores still do provide a delivery service and the order may be phoned in and delivered. Many housewives balk at this indulgence and worry about what it may cost. It may cost a little more but nothing to compare with the extra treatment that may be required for persistent recurrence of symptoms, and the unnecessary pain!

Sport and headaches

Exercise has a relaxing effect on most people especially if it is a sport which they enjoy. If the sport is very competitive the concomitant stress may bring on headache. Also the jarring of certain sports like squash could provoke headache. These factors will apply individually to each patient and she should be guided by her own tolerance.

15
Caution and contraindications

Although a great many conditions constitute contraindications to forceful (Grade V) manipulative technique, few preclude the use of the gentle controlled oscillatory pressures taught by Maitland.

Fortunately, in the case of cervical headaches most are totally relieved by means of the gentle technique. Occasionally, as is also the case in problems arising from other vertebral levels, the condition will improve on the gentle treatment to a certain level and then plateau. At this point it might become necessary to increase the strength of the technique to a Grade V in order to finally free the joint of restriction into the end of its range. When this situation presents, it is advisable to go back to the initial assessment and check for indications of the following conditions, which might preclude the use of forced movement.

1. Carcinoma with bony metastasis. This could have been suggested by a recent and significant loss of weight or by a history of surgery for cancer, e.g. mastectomy.
2. Evidence of osteoporosis on radiological studies, or the presence of a condition where osteoporosis may ensue, e.g. advanced age, post-menopausal women or a history of steroid therapy.
3. Radiological evidence of excessive exostosis in the region to be treated.
4. Neurological deficit arising from that area.
5. Instability of intervertebral joints in the region to be manipulated, whether due to fractures, subluxations or dislocations or unstable congenital anomalies.
6. Rheumatoid arthritis. (Even the gentlest mobilizing techniques should not be applied to the upper cervical spine.)
7. Protective muscle spasm. Never force through it.
8. Vertebral artery insufficiency. This could have been suggested in the subjective examination by reports of dizziness related to rotation or extension of the neck.

In the presence of the foregoing conditions, with the exception of rheumatoid arthritis, gentle oscillating technique may be used. It is essential that the therapist has a thorough appreciation of every aspect of the condition he is treating. The foregoing conditions would influence his choice of technique and the strength with which it is to be applied. Within these constraints he will be able to give the patient much relief.

Whether or not the patient complains of dizziness, it is wise to include in the objective examination a test for vertebral artery insufficiency. In the rare event of a patient having an abnormal vascular supply to the basilar artery system, she would be susceptible to injury which could occur during the performance of a manipulation that involves rotation or extension of the neck. The result could be fatal (Green and Joynt, 1959).

Vertebral artery patency tests

With the patient in a sitting position, ask her to turn her head to one side as far as she is able. The therapist holds her head in that position for about 15 seconds, then releases his hold and asks the patient how she feels. If this procedure causes the patient to feel dizzy, faint or nauseous, or if sensory or visual disturbance or nystagmus should result, the test is positive and no rotational, extension or forceful movement should be attempted. The test should be carried out to both the left and the right side.

If the result of the test is not clear, the same test is applied, only this time moving the head into extension and holding it there, and for even more certainty into a movement which combines extension, lateral flexion and rotation. These positions are held for 15 seconds and reassessed in the same way as described in the rotation test. These tests should be repeated with the patient lying supine.

In order to exclude the middle ear as the cause of dizziness one could do a test with the patient standing up, holding her head steady and asking her to rotate her body to each side. Dizziness provoked thus would exclude the middle ear as a cause because the semicircular canal fluid would not be disturbed by this test.

These tests should form a routine part of the objective examination so that the risk, small though it is, of vascular accident to the brainstem will be further minimized. Do not, however, rely too much on a negative test. I recall a patient whom I was treating for headache who had a long-standing history of severe dizziness, but in whom none of the aforementioned tests provoked dizziness. Because dizziness was the dominant symptom I sent him back to the doctor who ordered an angiogram. This demonstrated a complete shut-down of the right vertebral artery which was corrected surgically, after which the dizziness abated.

Another case which could have ended unhappily involved a middle-aged woman who presented with headache and a very stiff neck. Because she responded only marginally to the initial gentle mobilization and the stiffness seemed to require more forceful technique, I was about to carry out a Grade V rotation. I paused to test the vertebral artery, and while I was holding her head rotated to the left she slipped from my grasp and slid, unconscious, to the floor. She came to as I saved her head from hitting the floor.

Such cases are rare and I have only come across a few in the course of many years of practice. Nevertheless, the consequences can be so serious that the few minutes needed to test the patency of the vertebral arteries and to assess the extent of subjective reports of dizziness are well spent.

Congenital anomalies of the cervical spine should also be considered (Garber, 1964) and the therapist must be alert for complications that they might introduce.

Be alert for clues to serious pathology. Features which suggest serious intracranial pathology include:

1. Change in character of a chronic headache or an increase in severity.
2. Pain worst on waking in the morning or pain which wakes the patient at night.
3. Pain worsened by exertion, cough, sneeze or straining, positional change, movements and jolts.

4. Pain associated with vomiting, neurological symptoms or signs, e.g. seizures, confusion, depressed consciousness, ataxia, diplopia, papilloedema, focal signs or nuchal rigidity.
5. Non-specific character, severity and location of pain.

Sudden recent onset and rapid development of a syndrome could suggest intracranial pathology. Neck rigidity suggests meningitis. Some patients report that their headaches date from meningitis some years back. The cause of the headache in that case would be residual or progressive stiffness of the cervical joints following the inflammatory condition associated with neck rigidity. Mobilization would be appropriate treatment.

Most of the symptoms listed above are frequently associated with the advanced cervical headache syndrome, but in the presence of such symptoms, where the patient has not been neurologically investigated, the therapist should request such examination before proceeding with treatment.

Unusual responses

When there is an unusual or adverse response to the treatment this should also be reported to and discussed with the doctor. Exacerbation of pain after initial or subsequent treatment which was too vigorous does not constitute an adverse response. The fact that the pain is flared up in response to manipulative treatment is encouraging when one is seeking confirmation of a tentative diagnosis of a cervical mechanical cause for the headaches. The exacerbation from over-treatment of the craniovertebral joints is often alarmingly violent and lasts for longer than such an exacerbation does in lower vertebral levels. So if a patient with a long-standing and severe syndrome reports 'the worst headache she has ever had' following a treatment, it is not necessarily cause for alarm. One should reassure her and tell her that that was a good reaction and that subsequent treatment will not cause a repeat of the flare-up but will in all probability have increasingly positive results. To provoke a flare-up of pain is more encouraging than to provoke no response at all. But because this is so, the therapist should not seek to provoke this reaction. He should initially treat all headache cases as if the causative condition were irritable, more so than the most irritable vertebral condition in other regions of the spine.

By an adverse response the author has in mind the provocation of violent pain that does not subside within 24 hours and where there is no subsequent relief, or the onset of symptoms which were not present initially, such as dizziness, nausea, visual loss, ataxia or syncope. Also when there is no response at all, whatever strategy is applied to the cervical spine.

Sensory disturbances are common concomitants of cervical headache syndromes and do not in themselves constitute cause for alarm. But sensory aberrations which do not come and go with the headache should be reported as these might need to be investigated.

A headache case which presents without previous history of chronic headache but came on together with an acute torticollis could be expected to abate when the torticollis is reduced by means of Grade V manipulation if this is the treatment of choice as indicated by assessment. It should be the only time when a headache case is so strongly manipulated at the first visit, and should also only be done if contraindications to forceful technique have been excluded. If the initial assessment of the patient's condition is hastily done it will be inadequate for the purpose of picking up the important detail necessary to ensure the patient's safety.

References

Garber, J. N. (1964) Abnormalities of the atlas and axis vertebrae – congenital and traumatic. *Journal of Bone and Joint Surgery*, **46A**, 1782

Green, D. and Joynt, R. J. (1959) Vascular accidents to the brainstem associated with a neck manipulation. *Journal of the American Medical Association*, **170**, 522–524

Further reading

Maitland, G. D. (1986) *Vertebral Manipulation*, 5th edn pp. 182–185. Butterworths, London

Manipulative Therapists Association of Australia (1988) Protocol for premanipulative testing. *Australian Journal of Physiotherapy*, **34(2)**, 97–100

Orthopaedic Manipulative Therapist's Group (1991) Protocol for premanipulative testing. *South African Journal of Physiotherapy*, **47(1)**, 15–17

16

Case histories

In recording the treatment given the following symbols have been used: c/o, patient complains of; o/e, objective examination; // separates the description of the techniques applied from the assessed response of the patient.

Case 1

A middle-aged man, otherwise healthy and strong, complained of severe occipital headache. It had begun about 12 years previously following an incident where he had bumped his head on an overhead iron structure in a mine. Prior to that he had never experienced headache of any kind.

The headache had worsened over this period, becoming more severe and more frequent until it was continuous, which it had been for many years at the time of presentation.

P = 5/5

The intensity of pain fluctuated in that it was mild for half an hour to an hour in the mornings and then became severe for the rest of the day. About twice a month it became so bad that he felt blinded and unable to walk.

I = 5/5

He described it as a throbbing pain with a feeling of pressure. When the pain was severe he took two Syndol (an analgesic compound), which lessened the pain but did not take it away. He took Syndol every day. Previously he had used Codis (a simple analgesic) which initially took the pain away for a short while but later, when it became less effective, he changed to Syndol.

R = 4/5
TPP = 14/15

Aggravating and precipitating factors were: car travel, reading, watching television, working with his neck bent to one side, lifting a weight of 15–20kg (e.g. a chair or a box of cold drinks) which is not a heavy weight for him. He was not able to partake of wine or beer at all because it resulted in severe headache, but whisky taken in milk eased the pain. When the pain was severe he was unable to read because the letters moved. He also saw small spots, heard a zooming sound in his ears, felt nauseous, dizzy, 'drunk in the head' and felt pins and needles in his left fingers.

Previous examination had included X-rays of the neck which, he told me, showed three lesions. (The X-rays had been taken many years earlier and were not available.) He had then been referred for physiotherapy for his overtly cervical problem. He said that he had derived no relief at all from the physiotherapy (pre-Maitland heat and massage). He had then gone to a chiropractor and his manipulation caused the headache to abate for a year. When he returned he got less relief than he did the first time round and when he returned for a third lot of treatment from the chiropractor he obtained no relief at all. He had resorted to self-administered pain killers and had used them daily for years. His health, apart from the low blood pressure, was good. As a child he had not suffered motion sickness nor had he been an allergic child. There was no family history of chronic headache.

His doctor referred him to me for 'five treatments of physiotherapy to his neck'.

On examination

Now: c/o – Mild occipital pain spreading to the vertex.

Neck – bilateral soreness and stiffness suboccipital to tip of shoulder area, also central at level C7.

Active physiological movement

Flexion: full range and no increase of pain with overpressure.
Extension: full range and no increase of pain with overpressure, but neck pain came on after maintaining the overpressure for a few seconds.
Left and right side flexion: full range but neck pain increased with overpressure.
Left rotation: full range with latent pain after maintained overpressure.
Right rotation: full range and no pain increase with maintained overpressure.

The patency of the vertebral artery was tested because of the subjective complaint of dizziness with severe headache but was found not to be compromised.

Passive accessory intervertebral movement testing by palpation

This revealed tenderness on central postero-anterior pressure on the arch of the atlas on a Grade II pressure, and also, bilaterally, on the articular pillar at C2 level with the head in neutral position and also with the head in rotation. Stiffness and tenderness were also palpated bilaterally at all cervical levels to various extents.

Treatment

Central vertebral pressure on C1	// c/o
5 × Grade II pressures	// Vertex pain has gone
(because of the vertex pain)	//
Unilateral vertebral pressures	//
on C2 (C2/C3 joint) 5 × Grade II	//
pressures on the left and on	//
the right	//
and	
Unilateral vertebral pressures	//
on C2 with the head turned first	//
to the left and then to the	//
right (C1/C2 joint) 7 × Grade II	// c/o
pressures on each side	// Occipital pain has gone

Stiff and tender lower cervical joints (because of the neck pain) were mobilized with Grade II unilateral vertebral pressures, about 20 pressures to each.
Note: The treatments given to levels O/C1/C2 were specifically aimed at the head pain. When that had cleared, the neck pain was attended to.
Massage and ultrasound was then given to reduce the considerable cervical muscle spasm.

At his next visit three days later he said that two hours after the first treatment the headache resumed with alarming severity. Then it subsided gradually and finally was quite gone and he had not felt it since. The treatment on that day was a repeat of that given on the first day but the number of pressures was increased to 20 each because, although initial mobilization resulted in an exacerbation of symptoms, the latent effect was favourable. Also the joint tenderness was so much less on Grade II pressures that it was decided to increase the number of pressures substantially rather than increase the grade of pressure.

At his next appointment two days later, he reported no recurrence of headache but said that his neck felt a little stiff. The previous treatment was repeated and the patient was asked to return after a week.

When he returned he said that he had had no headache during that week and that his neck felt fine. The treatment was repeated and he was discharged and asked to return only if and when there was a recurrence. Neck movements should have been retested but as the spontaneous reports of improvement were so positive, this was not clinically necessary.

Ten months later he returned and told us that the headache had stayed away for nine months but had been building up again over the previous month and he was then having headache again every night and whenever he lifted heavy objects. On palpation there was tenderness again centrally on C1 but only on a Grade IV pressure, and also pain and stiffness at the C1/2 level on Grade II pressure.

(Compare this with the initial assessment at first presentation. This increased tolerance of passive accessory movement indicates an improvement in the joint condition, which is borne out by the considerable de-escalation of the syndrome as it was then.)

Before commencement of this treatment he had suboccipital pain and neck pain.

Treatment

Central postero-anterior vertebral	
pressures on C1, Grade IV × 5	//
and bilateral postero-anterior	//
vertebral pressures on C2 with the	//
head rotated first left and then right	// c/o
Grade II × 10 pressures	// No pain now

On the following day he reported that there had been no recurrence of headache but that the neck felt stiff. The treatment aimed at the headache on the previous day was repeated and the neck mobilized, after which he said that the neck no longer felt stiff. He was again discharged, to report recurrence.

Seven months later he returned. He reported that he had not been troubled with headache since the last visit. On closer questioning he said that he had had very occasional headaches, less frequently than once a month, that they had been mild and had gone away when he took one Disprin.

TPP = 3/15 (P = 1/5, I = 1/5, R = 1/5)

He had returned, not because of headache but because his neck had gradually stiffened and become painful over the past week. He complained that turning his neck produced a pain reaching from the right upper region of the neck to the spine of the scapula and that if he tried to lift more than 25 kg the neck pain radiated into the head.

On examining his physiological cervical movement

It was found that:

On extending the neck in the ordinary way, he had a full range of movement with pain only coming in when overpressure was applied. But he pointed out that if he tightened his neck and then extended it he could go no more than 1/4 range before the whole extent of the neck–scapular pain increase markedly. (This was consistent with the pain being brought on while lifting.) Left side flexion was painful when overpressure was applied but right side flexion was limited to 1/4 range and this produced the same neck–scapular pain.

On palpation over the right articular pillar there was no pain and stiffness over the C and C7 levels but after mobilizing these joints, using Grade III pressures, there was still the same pain when he extended his neck with tightened muscles, but perhaps a little less severe. Because there were no contraindications to a more forceful technique, his neck was manipulated with a transverse thrust, Grade V, towards the right, localized to C7. Ice and ultrasound were then applied.

When he returned the following day he reported a difference 'like night and day'. The same treatment was repeated on that day. He was seen again five days later, when his neck movements were of full range and pain-free, and he had had no neck pain or headache. Localized manipulation, Grade V, was carried out at C2 and C7 and the patient was again discharged to report recurrences, which he has not done to date (six months later).

The self-help advice to this patient was to avoid lifting even what, to him, are light weights. I do not think that the condition will recur regularly and if it does, one or two treatments a couple of times a year is to be preferred to the regular use of drugs.

Note: His headache, which had been continuous for years at a TPP = 13/15 had now been reduced to a level of TPP = 3/15, which is an acceptable syndrome to most people. They would not seek medical help for it. They would perceive it to be normal, and think that most people have such a headache on occasion.

Case 2

A middle-aged woman, otherwise healthy, presented with frontal and occipital pain which at times radiated down the right side of the neck and also, at times, down the right arm to her fingers. Her right ear sometimes felt dead and as if there was pressure there. She said that usually the head pain could be described as an ache, but at times when it became severe there was a feeling of such pressure that it felt as if her head would burst. The pain would then be so severe that she could not remain on her feet and was obliged to lie down.

I = 5/5

The headaches had begun ten years before after she had had a hysterectomy. Prior to this she had never known headache at all. Two years later she had sustained a whiplash injury in a motor collision. The condition had worsened over this period of time. Previously the intensity of pain had not been prostrating, and it was intermittent, its presence increasing until it became continuous, which it had been for five days at the time of presentation.

P = 5/5

Simple analgesics had no effect on the pain and Voltaren (an anti-inflammatory compound) eased it but did not cause it to abate. She was using about 30 Voltaren per month.

R = 4/5
TPP = 14/15

The headache was aggravated by noisy music, car lights when driving at night (cervical muscle tension resulting from irritation), when she became cross (adrenaline-induced cervical muscle contraction), although when she cried the headache lessened (presumably because of a tension release). When she sewed her neck pain, but not necessarily her headache, increased.

When the headache was severe she felt nauseous, had epigastric pain and since the headache had worsened and become continuous for the past several days, she had begun to see spots before her eyes. She also experienced dizziness when rising from a bent position.

She did not consult a doctor when the headaches started after the hysterectomy. (They were not yet as severe as they later became.) After the whiplash injury eight years before, she had seen a doctor who had prescribed physiotherapy for the neck injury. According to her clinical notes, taken by my junior physiotherapist, this treatment 'helped for a time'. This does not tell us whether there was an improvement in the headache syndrome or whether it was the early post-traumatic neck symptoms which were temporarily relieved and so is not a useful piece of information.

However, the headache must have resumed because the patient was later sent to an orthopaedic surgeon who diagnosed a disc lesion at level C5/6 and sent the patient to another physiotherapist who administered traditional physiotherapy which 'did not help at all'.

When she returned to her doctor still complaining of an ever worsening headache, he referred her to an ear, nose and throat specialist to investigate the possibility of a headache caused by sinusitis. Tests were negative.

After a long period she sought the advice of another doctor hoping to find relief for the headache which had by now become more than she could bear (**TPP = 14/15**). This doctor referred her to us with a script which read 'Osteoarthritis neck. Disc lesion C5/6'.

This patient had been a car-sick child and motion sick on roundabouts. She was allergic to penicillin. There was no family history of chronic headache.

On examination

Now: Right-sided temporal pain radiating back over the vertex and down the neck towards the right shoulder.
(Physiological movements were not tested, but should have been because neck pain was present.)

Passive accessory intervertebral movement testing by palpation

Unilateral postero-anterior vertebral pressure, C1 on the right, both close to the tubercle and midway between the tubercle and the extremity of the arch, were found to be tender to Grade II pressures.

Unilateral postero-anterior vertebral pressure on the right, over the articular pillar at C2 and C3, C5 and C7 levels were also painful on Grade II pressures.

Treatment

5 × Grade II pressures to each painful articulation, after which ice and ultrasound were administered // There was no noticeable change of symptoms

The patient was allowed to go home to return the following day and to notice relevant changes in the pain pattern.

On the following day she reported a significant flare-up of headache, severe enough to make her lie down.

Now: A dull right-sided frontal ache spreading down to the neck. The right cheek felt very tender.

The treatment of the previous day was repeated exactly (because of the flare-up) and after that she said that the pain was less.

At her next visit two days later, after a weekend, she said that her headache had not been too bad over the weekend (I would have liked this report to be more explicit, e.g. how much time with pain, how much without and compare it with the previous few days). However, on that Monday morning on waking there had been no pain (compare with the foregoing week or so when there was continuous pain).

Now: Light headache and cervical pain

Treatment

Repeat previous day's treatment // All pain has gone

Note: Although this pain responded promptly to each treatment, it took seventeen treatments over a period of two months before the syndrome was quite halted. There had also been some complaint of low back pain and arm pain, so it was complex in that it was a multiple joint condition. These complaints were also dealt with but are not transcribed here.

Seven and a half months later the patient returned with a recurrence of the headache which started up again after a difficult tooth extraction when the dentist had struggled for 20 minutes before the tooth came away.

The headache had been continuous for the fortnight since the dental work.

P = 5/5

The intensity of pain was disabling as it had been before.

I = 5/5

There was a poor response to analgesics.

R = 4/5

TPP = 14/15

She again saw spots and heard the ringing in her ears. She had consumed 100 pain killers in the past two weeks.

But although the symptom syndrome seemed to be as bad as it had been at first presentation, it only took five treatments to get it under control this time.

Discussion

This case portrays a typical natural history of the development of a cervical headache in that it began with some sort of trauma and worsened over the years until it became continuous.

The causative injury is more often a blow to the head or a whiplash injury but it is not uncommon for a patient undergoing any procedure under general anaesthetic to sustain, while anaesthetized, a joint lesion, vertebral or peripheral. This is probably due to inexpert handling during transfers when the patient's protective mechanisms are not operative and joints are overstretched or placed in abnormal postures and so maintained until the patient awakes and takes over control of her joints.

There was, however, a repeated frank trauma two years later which contributed to the escalation of the condition of late post-traumatic osteoarthritis. The recurrence after a prolonged dental session is of interest and highlights the causative trauma.

Another interesting feature is the fact that a few well-directed passive movements of the culpable joint instantly abated a pain which responded poorly or not at all to compound analgesics.

Case 3

A 37-year-old woman presented with frontal headache which was sometimes more severe over the left eye and sometimes over the right. There was no pain anywhere else in the head nor did her neck ever hurt.

It was a continuous ache but two or three times a week she was incapacitated.

P = 5/5

She had experienced what she called normal headache for many years, but 12 weeks ago the normal headache had worsened alarmingly in severity and had become continuous. She could remember no relevant trauma.

I = 5/5

She was taking 12 pain tablets per day, and whatever she tried was only partially effective, reducing the pain briefly but not causing it to abate. There was no difference in the effect of analgesics and migraine-specific drugs.

R = 4/5

TPP = 14/15

The pain intensity was aggravated by loud noise, stress (especially anger) and car travel. There were no associated symptoms.

She had first consulted her general practitioner who diagnosed a tension headache and prescribed relaxant drugs. These had no effect. A friend then suggested she visit a chiropractor and then an acupuncturist and again there was no response at all. She returned to her doctor and he ordered X-rays of her neck from which no abnormality could be detected.

She was then sent to a neurosurgeon where the condition was thoroughly investigated. Lumbar puncture, a brain scan, an electrocardiograph and blood tests revealed no relevant pathology and the neurosurgeon made a tentative diagnosis of migraine and prescribed suitable medication. This, too, proved to be ineffective.

She had been a motion-sick child but not allergic and there was no family history of chronic headache.

She was eventually sent to us by her general practitioner with a referral which read: 'Mrs —— has headache – fully investigated – N.A.D. I am sure these are tension (muscle contraction) headaches. Could you please give the necessary physiotherapy.'

On examination

My assistant who assessed and treated this case did not test cervical physiological movement because there was no neck pain. If she had I would have expected these movements to have been of full range and pain-free.

However, on palpating for accessory intervertebral movement, marked tenderness was found to be present along the atlanto-occipital junction on Grade II pressures. Postero-anterior unilateral vertebral pressure, Grade II, on the transverse processes of C2 was also tender.

Immediately before the first trial technique it was established that the headache was present and recorded thus:

Now: Frontal headache.

Treatment

Postero-anterior vertebral pressures	//
centrally and bilaterally on the arch of the	//
atlas with the head flexed fully on the	//
neck, rotating the head slightly and	// c/o No effect
progressively to the left and to the right	
(*see* Chapter 10)	//
Grade II × 10 at each point	//
Unilateral postero-anterior	//
vertebral pressures on the left	// c/o Pain intensity
and on the right on C2,	// slightly less and is now
Grade II × 10 to each side	// stronger over the right
	// eye
Transverse unilateral vertebral	//
pressures C1, Grade II × 5	// c/o Pain slightly less
pressures to each side	// intense over right eye

On the following day she said that the pain had become worse after the treatment for a few hours but had then decreased to below its usual level until bedtime. Then it was bad again and she took two pain tablets. On waking this morning it was more severe than yesterday morning.

Now: Frontal headache worse than this time yesterday and worse over the left eye.

Treatment

Postero-anterior pressures
on the arch of the atlas as
yesterday, Grade II × 10 to
each point
	//
	//
	// c/o Frontal pain slightly
	// less

Postero-anterior central vertebral pressure on C2 in a cephalad direction, Grade II × 10	// // c/o No change //

Postero-anterior central and
bilateral vertebral pressures
on C3, Grade II × 10 to each
	//
	// c/o Headache decidedly
	// lessened

On the following day the patient said that after the previous day's treatment the pain remained less than usual till about six o'clock that evening when it again became severe. She took two tablets and the pain lessened, which was the usual effect.

Now: Frontal headache but less severe than yesterday at this time.

This patient did not show dramatic improvement from day to day as we have come to expect with these cases, but the response to treatment each time was sufficient to make my assistant persevere. She was assessed and treated along the lines indicated with small daily gains, but this case was unusual because the improvement achieved was only in the pain intensity whereas the periodicity remained constant. After eight treatments over a period of two weeks, my assistant asked me to review the case. The patient said that the headaches were continuous but at a low level, specifically, that the level of the constant pain was less than it had been before commencing treatment and that she no longer had the exacerbations that she was having two or three times a week. She had not needed to take pain tablets for four days (compare 12 tablets per day before commencement of treatment).

I varied the treatment again, using an anterior approach to the upper cervical paravertebral joints, increased the grades and attempted, after checking on the vertebral artery patency, localized manipulation (Grade V) but muscle spasm prevented an effective Grade V. Overall there was as usual after the previous treatments a lessening of the present pain but nothing that I could think of doing abated the pain even briefly. I then incorporated traction (upper cervical) 10 lb for 10 minutes together with a hot pack under the neck, and also instruction on relaxation and de-contraction of the neck muscles. After nine more such treatments, using Grade III and IV techniques, and an occasional Grade V localized to the O/C1/C2 levels followed by traction, she was discharged to report progress or otherwise. At this stage the periodicity was still 5/5 but because the intensity was so low (I = 1/5 and only occasionally 2/5), and she no longer needed pain tablets, it was decided to stop treatment as we did not think that she would improve further. She was quite prepared to accept this situation and said that she was able to do whatever she wanted to do and was not hampered by the slight pain.

Two months later she phoned to tell us that the headache was still ever present but hovered between 1–/5 and 1+/5 and that she had not had anything more severe than that. She also was happy that she had travelled to Durban by car for a short holiday and had not arrived there with a worse headache such as had always been the case in the past.

Her TPP is now maintained, despite the ever presence of the headache, at:

P = 5/5
I = 1/5
R = 0
TPP = 6/15

compared to the initial **TPP = 14/15**

(*see Figure 12.3*)

(R in such cases is difficult to assess, but as she is not needing or using analgesia it is irrelevant.)

Case 4

A 36-year-old man presented with occipital pain occupying the occiput from the vertex to the nuchal line. He had occasional neck pain with movement and sometimes felt a stabbing pain in the neck even while sitting still.

He said that he had had headaches since childhood. For a long time he had occasional headache, roughly once a month, and then they came more frequently and for the previous year they had come twice a week until two months ago when the headache had become continuous.

P = 5/5

The intensity of pain, although quite bad at times, was not disabling and he was able to continue with his work.

I = 3/5

Initially a patent painkiller had taken the pain away but over the years had become less effective until the time came when it had no effect at all. Now the tablets he had on his doctor's prescription slightly lessened the pain.

R = 5/5
TPP = 13/15

When questioned about relevant trauma he remembered that he had fallen backwards out of a tree onto his head at the age of 12.

Aggravating and precipitating factors were: sharp light, performing heavy physical work, driving if he does not sit in precisely the right posture, everyday tensions and immediately whenever he flexes his neck.

Associated symptoms were dizziness (especially when he had done any work involving neck flexion), black moving dots before his eyes, epigastric pain (but, he says he had a hiatus hernia) and just recently the pain was accompanied by nausea.

While his headaches were intermittent he had never sought medical help. But when they became continuous, he consulted his doctor, a general practitioner. The doctor diagnosed a headache due to hypertension and prescribed treatment to bring his blood pressure under control. He also gave him 'pills for rheumatism', but this treatment regime did not alter the headache and so he went to another doctor who diagnosed a cervical problem and referred him to us for physiotherapy.

This patient had once become nauseous when he went on too many roundabouts at a fair, but otherwise was not motion sick as a child and nor had he been an allergic child. There was no family history of chronic headache.

On examination

All cervical physiological movements caused neck pain at the end of range.

Passive accessory intervertebral movement testing by palpation

Unilateral postero-anterior vertebral pressure on the articular pillar at level C2 was painful on Grade II pressure, both on the left and on the right sides.

Now: Vertex, occipital and nuchal pain.

Treatment

Unilateral postero-anterior pressure at C2 level, left and right, Grade II × 15 pressures	// c/o No change in the headache
Unilateral antero-posterior pressures on C2, left and right, Grade II × 15 pressures	// c/o Headache shortened towards the neck Now only suboccipital

However on leaving the pain was again back to the vertex – the full extent as it had been before. He was sent home and asked to note any change in the pattern that he had described.

The following day he reported that three hours after the previous day's treatment the headache had become more severe and had remained so until the present.

Now: The pain was present in the same distribution as the day before but more severe.

Trial traction applied manually with the patient supine had no effect on the pain. Mobilization of the temporomandibular joint, although painful, also had no effect. Unilateral postero-anterior pressure on C1 at the point where palpation was most tender, Grade IV × 10 pressures to both left and right sides, had no effect on the headache. Unilateral postero-anterior vertebral pressures on C2 with the head in rotation, first to the left and then to the right, Grade IV × 10 also did not decrease the pain or change its distribution in any way, but after that his eyes were 'pulsating'.

The technique described on page 109, where the whole extent of the border between the atlas and the skull is deeply palpated whilst progressively rotating the head, revealed tender areas but mobilization of this joint, Grade IV × 10, had no effect.

The patient was then given traction with the upper cervical spine in the neutral position, 20 lb rhythmic, and ice therapy to the upper neck.

Because the headache so stubbornly failed to respond to so many techniques applied to what I thought were the culpable joints, I precipitately returned the patient to the doctor for further investigation.

The doctor referred the patient to the orthopaedic surgeon who sent him back to us and said that we had not tried hard enough.

My junior assistant reassessed the condition and found that the periodicity had improved: it was now intermittent and so rated a P = 4/5 where it had been P = 5/5. The intensity was still 3/5 and he had stopped taking tablets (no reason given).

Now: Vertex pain, no occipital pain.

The therapist palpated extra thoroughly and found that central and unilateral postero-anterior vertebral pressure on both sides of C1 were very tender and twice gave 5 × Grade III pressures at each site, and the headache lessened after each volley of 5 but did not abate. He then mobilized C2 centrally, moving the spinous process in a cephalad direction, but the headache was still there, though less severe when the patient went home.

On the following day the patient reported that the headache remained less severe for only ten minutes after leaving before becoming worse than before that treatment and remained worse until he went to bed. On waking this morning the pain was less than usual in the morning.

Now: Vertex pain.

Treatment exactly as on the previous day was given, with some resultant fluctuation of pain, worse and then less pain after each technique, and he left with the vertex pain less than when he came in.

On the following day he said that the pain had remained less for three hours after the previous treatment and then again had become worse than usual. On waking it was as usual on waking.

Now: Slight vertex pain.

The treatment was carried out as on the previous day, but 10 of each pressure were given. There was no response at all now.

After more palpation she found that if she placed her thumbs on the superior aspect of the spinous process of C2 and moved it in a caudad direction, the headache lessened. She repeated three volleys of 10 × Grade III pressures in this manner and when he left he said that the headache had nearly gone.

On the next day he reported that the headache had gone completely after he left for some hours, and that when it had returned it was very mild, and that it came and went, but always very mildly until:

Now: Very slight vertex pain.

After repeating the last-mentioned technique only, using Grade III × 10, that pain was gone.

The patient needed only one more treatment, and only the last technique was used, and his headache syndrome abated.

Case 5

A 58-year-old woman was plagued by right-sided parietal headache which seemed to stem from a circumscribed area at the base of the skull and encroached on the right temple and maxilla. The pain throbbed at times and she had a feeling of pressure 'like a tight hat'.

The headache occurred on three or four days a week,

P = 3/5

when it was so severe that she was obliged to sit or lie down. She said that when it was so bad she could stay on her feet but that she was unable to do anything and couldn't bear to speak to anyone.

I = 5/5

As a young child she had suffered from ear trouble which was accompanied by headache which at times prevented her from attending school. These headaches continued into adulthood but had only become so frequent during the past year. They had also become much more severe than ever before. In February 1983 she had fallen and hit her head on a step. She said that she was unconscious, but only briefly. In July 1983 she had had a cerebral haemorrhage drained. She said that her headaches had started to become worse since then.

R = 4+/5

She took one pain tablet only when the pain was very bad, and if she then lay down the pain would ease a bit but not go away. She used about five pain tablets per week. She was also on medication for hypertension. She is allergic to aspirin.

Bright lights hurt her eyes and resulted in headache. Other aggravating or precipitating factors were: watching television or reading which also made her eyes burn, hard work, e.g. gardening, or becoming annoyed or emotionally upset.

When the pain was severe she felt dizzy and had very brief blank spells. Tiny coloured lights moved across her field of vision and there was tinnitus which sounded like birds twittering and sometimes like a telephone ringing. There was epigastric pain with the headache and globulus hystericus, and she said that it was difficult to swallow her saliva.

Previous treatment had been medication, but because she was allergic to aspirin this posed a problem.

On examination

Cervical physiological movement

Flexion – Right suboccipital pain increased at full range.
Extension – Full range, left trapezius pain on overpressure.
Left flexion – Pain right side neck at 3/4 range.
Right flexion – Pain left side neck just before end of range.
Left rotation – Full range, right neck and left trapezius pain with overpressure.
Right rotation – Full range, right side neck pain.

Palpation of accessory intervertebral movement

Transverse vertebral pressure against the tip of the transverse process of C1 on the right was tender to Grade I pressure, as was right unilateral postero-anterior vertebral pressure on the articular pillar at level C2.

Now: Right-sided parietal pain extending down the right side of the neck.

Treatment

Transverse vertebral pressures	//	
against the tip of the transverse	//	
process of C1 directed from the	//	c/o The parietal pain has
right towards the left,	//	gone
Grade I × 5 pressures	//	
Unilateral postero-anterior pressures	//	
on the articular pillar on	//	c/o Neck pain feels better
the right at level C2, Grade I	//	o/e All movements
× 10 pressures	//	improved

D + 1

When she got home after the previous day's treatment, the right parietal and neck pain became worse, that is, much worse than it had been before. She rested and the pain then went away without having taken any tablets, which was unusual. This morning, after an emotional upset right-sided headache came on, also right-sided sternal pain.

Now: Right parietal pain

Treatment

Previous day's treatment repeated exactly. As this patient was also referred for lumbar pain, this was also assessed and treated on this day (not reproduced here)

Note: Cervical physiological movements, although tested on the first day, were not retested because adequate subjective information for the purpose of reassessment was forthcoming. If this had not been the case and this headache had turned out to be a poor responder, the record of the objective tests would have been useful, as one of the things one might need to do in that case would be to work at eliminating these signs and aiming at a full pain-free range of movement.

D + 2

The back pain was gone after treatment and had returned but only slightly that morning. The patient was surprised at this prompt response and said that she could hardly believe it. The headache and neck pain, however, was 'terribly painful' after treatment as on the day before and there was a burning feeling in the neck, but she had woken this morning with no pain at all in the head or neck and later felt a 'dull streaky ache' in the right side of the head and neck.

Now: Has pain in the tip of the right scapula and slight low back pain.

Treatment

The treatment as given for head and neck pain on the previous two days was repeated, with the addition of:

Unilateral postero-anterior pressures on the articular pillar at level C7 on the right, Grade III × 2 minutes (for scapula tip pain)

Note: The treatment of the head and neck pain was repeated exactly because it was being effective. However it was not increased because it caused a considerable pain increase each time before subsequent relief.

D + 3

Woke in the night with pain behind the left ear radiating down the left side of the neck (contralateral to the usual distribution of pain: this can indicate improvement in the condition). It went away after taking a pain tablet. The right-sided pain had not returned.

Now: Scapular pain and dull backache.

Treatment

The previous day's treatment was repeated with an increase in the grade and number of pressures applied

D + 7

She said that she 'felt great' after the previous treatment and was even able to garden without the usual ill effect. She had woken in the night with head pain but it had soon gone away. The low back pain had also shown further improvement and was now 'only a small ache'.

Now: Left high parietal pain.
Low backache.

Treatment

Transverse vertebral pressures on C1 towards the left and towards the right, Grade II × 20 pressures

Unilateral postero-anterior vertebral pressures on the articular pillar at levels C2 and C7, Grade IV × 20 pressures to each

Treatment for lumbar spine

The next visit, two days later, the patient said that she was much better in that her head, neck, scapular and lumbar pain were subsiding. The previous treatment was repeated and the patient was asked to return in a week and to report on the behaviour of all pain.

One week later she reported that she had been well and doing a lot more than she had been able to do before presentation. But on this morning there had been a recurrence of pain.

Now: Right occipital pain
Right scapular pain, sharp
Lumbar pain on the right

After repeating the treatment given on the previous day all the pain listed above had abated.

Seven more treatments were needed and the treatment was increased in strength to Grade IV pressures and the number of pressures increased. The headache seemed to have abated and she was discharged and asked to report recurrences.

This case was followed up two years later when she said that headaches were no longer a problem to her and that she hardly ever had a headache.

Case 6

A middle-aged woman presented with a very severe syndrome of headache. The pain radiated from the suboccipital area over the occiput as far as the vertex and also to both temples. The vertex and temple pain was sharp and burning. There was also a stabbing feeling in or behind the ears.

The pain intensity became intolerable and for two days prior to presentation she had been unable to sleep at all.

I = 5/5

The headache had been there continuously for two years at an intensity which fluctuated around I = 4/5.

P = 5/5

Prior to a 'nervous breakdown' five years before she had had 'normal headaches' ever since her childhood. But for the five years following the nervous breakdown the normal headaches had worsened, both in intensity of pain and frequency until they had become a continuous headache two years before.

Initially, any painkiller would take the pain away. Currently no analgesic had any effect on the pain.

R = 5/5

As a child she remembered slipping on a hard veranda and hitting her head. In 1975 (10 years before) she says that she had another bad fall.

Aggravating factors were: reducing the use of her 'nerve pills'; wine, especially champagne; sharp light, noise or 'when things are too quiet'; car travel – even around town – she is unable to do her shopping; when she cries or becomes angry. When she has been tense and under pressure, the pain gets worse afterwards when she relaxes.

Associated symptoms were: dizziness and fainting, loss of memory, epigastric pain, seeing stars, hearing buzzing noise most of the time, numbness in all fingers, paraesthesia of scalp and around mouth. She experienced nausea for the first time a few days before.

She had suffered nervous breakdown on four occasions and the last one, five years before, had been very bad. Electroencephalograms and brain CT scans showed no abnormality and the headache was diagnosed as a tension headache. No treatment was prescribed for the headache, although she had psychiatric treatment daily for three weeks. A cervical manipulation done by her general practitioner relieved the pain briefly but when this was repeated at a later stage, it had no effect. Another general practitioner had given hydrocortisone injections on five occasions. These helped for a year, then for lessening periods, and they were not repeated after the fifth time. By 'helped' it is meant that the headaches were less severe but did not abate.

Medication for her nervous condition was : Lexotan (tranquillizer) 6 mg 2×/day; Tofranil (CNS stimulant) 10 mg 2×/day; Premarin (oestrogen) 0.625 g; Trasicor (adrenergic beta-blocker) 1/day; and something else, the name of which she had forgotten.

There were no recent X-rays of her neck.

Note: It was not possible to make this assessment on the first day of presentation as the patient arrived in extreme pain and was unable to answer questions. My assistant wisely palpated for the likely source of pain, and finding the occipito-atlantal joint extremely tender whichever way it was approached, gave five Grade I pressures over the most tender areas.

Cervical physiological movement

Flexion: at less than half range there was an increase of upper cervical pain.

Extension: upper cervical pain increased at half range. Left and right side flexion, and left and right rotation also increased the same pain at half range.

Treatment

Postero-anterior unilateral vertebral pressures, on the left and on the right on C1, starting at the tubercle and moving laterally whilst progressively rotating the head (*see* Chapter 12)	
Five Grade I pressures at each most tender spot	
Also transverse vertebral pressures against the tip of the transverse process of C1, from the left and from the right, Grade I × 5	// c/o // The headache intensity is much less

On the following day the patient reported that the pain intensity had remained less, as it had become after the previous day's treatment, that she had slept well and assessed the pain intensity that morning at 3/5.

I = 3/5

The subjective assessment was then done and the pain present immediately prior to the ensuing treatment was assessed.

Now: Right-sided parietal pain only, dull. Upper cervical pain.

Treatment

Unilateral postero-anterior vertebral pressures along the arch of the atlas as on the previous day, Grade I × 5 to each tender point Also, unilateral postero-anterior pressures on the left and the right on C2–C7, Grade I × 10 to each (for the neck pain)	// c/o // The headache has gone

Also, because on palpation she was found to be tender lower down:
Unilateral postero-anterior vertebral pressures on the left and on the right on C7 and T1–T8, Grade II × 10 to each
	// c/o
	// Neck pain feels much
	// better

On the following day she reported that the headache had not come back for many hours, but that this morning the headache was quite severe. She had waited until noon and then taken two Disprin which had the effect of lessening the pain. Her neck felt more mobile.

Note: Initially she had reported that no analgesic had any effect on the pain and so this was an encouraging factor, R now 2/5 compared to 5/5.

Now: Bilateral parietal and right temporal pain. Neck feels tight again.

The treatment of the previous day was repeated exactly, after which she said that the headache was gone and also the neck symptoms.

On the next day she said that the headache had stayed away for 8 hours, but that it had returned this morning and was quite severe.

Now: Bilateral temporal and right-sided parietal pain and burning.

The treatment given the previous day to the O/C1/C2 joints was repeated and also transverse pressures on C1 towards the left and the right, Grade II × 5 to each side, after which the pain had gone again.

Her next visit was three days later, when she reported some headache on the day after treatment but no headache for the next two days.

Now: No headache.

Treatment was repeated as on the previous visit.
Next day: c/o still no headache.
Treatment was repeated as before.

Three days later there was still no headache and because she had had no pain for a week, she was treated as before and discharged and asked to report recurrence.

Three months later I telephoned her to follow-up the case. She said that she was very well and happy to be free of headache. When I asked her if she never had headache she said that on occasion, when she was under pressure, for example on a Monday when all her children had been to visit over the weekend and she had had an excess of housework and cooking to do, she would wake with a headache, but, she said, the intensity was about a quarter of what it had been before. But it presented no problem because my assistant had shown her how to perform the technique which relieved her headache. Whenever she felt the headache coming on, instead of taking a painkiller she treated herself as taught and had consistently been able to abort the headache. She had been given tablets by her doctor with instructions that, should this self-help fail, she was to take them and report at once for more of the same therapy, but this had not been necessary to date.

Case 7

I was asked by a neurosurgeon to see a 47-year-old woman in hospital for intractable headache. She had been admitted a week before for the headache which had become so severe that she could neither walk nor drive her car and was obliged to remain in bed. She had been unable to eat and had vomited for four days.

I = 5/5

The pain distribution was like a cap over the top of her head with shooting pains into the vertex and into either the left or the right temple, with a piercing stab into the ipsilateral eye. She also had neck pain, mainly upper cervical, which, she said felt as if her neck was broken. The neck pain was particularly painful when she extended it, for example, to kiss her husband.

The headache made her feel as if 'her eyes were out on stalks and her nose was about to bleed'. It was a throbbing pain and at times it felt as if her head would explode. Her neck felt stiff and extremely painful. The severity of the head pain varied from mild at times to very bad, so as to make her nauseous. When severe she was obliged to go home from work and lie down.

She had experienced occasional headaches since reaching adulthood, but these had become more frequent and during the year just passed were present on every second day. Sixteen weeks ago the headache had become continuous.

P = 5/5

It had worsened in intensity over the past two weeks, of which she had spent one week at home in bed and the second week in hospital.

The only relevant trauma that she could remember was that she had walked into a kitchen cupboard and hit her head – she had done this twice during the previous two years.

Analgesics which had relieved the pain before no longer had any effect. Before the headaches became so bad, Disprin was effective, and when they no longer gave relief she used Anadin and then Grandpa powders (another painkiller) until eventually none of these afforded any relief at all.

R = 5/5

TPP = 15/15

Factors that made her headache worse or brought it on when it was not there were: being tired or upset (she has her own shop and its day-to-day problems to do with labourers upset her), bright lights and noise, watching television (she had been obliged to give up watching television), driving any distance. Sometimes the headache woke her during the night.

When the pain was severe she felt nauseous and vomited. Her gait was also disturbed and she said that she 'misplaced steps'. She was dizzy and heard a ringing in her ears which sounded like Christmas beetles.

She had not consulted a doctor about the headache until it had escalated so badly and become continuous, and then she was hospitalized. In hospital, her neck was X-rayed and an electroencephalogram was carried out. X-ray showed a lesion at C6/7. She was given migraine tablets and tranquillizers, and sleeping tablets at night. Although there had not been even a brief remission of the pain the intensity was less while under this regimen, although for three of the days during the week in hospital it had been extremely severe. This was after the investigative procedures.

She had not been a motion-sick or an allergic child and there was no family history of chronic headache.

On examination

Before commencing the tests it was established that the headache was present. She said that the whole head was throbbing. The last drug taken had worn off and she was about to take another. Her neck was also sore and she complained of tinnitus.

Cervical physiological movement

Flexion: at half range, low cervical pain was felt.
Extension: full range, pulling feeling at the end.
Left flexion: contralateral neck pain at half range.
Right flexion: contralateral neck pain at half range.
Left and right rotation were of full range and pain-free with overpressure.

Palpation of intervertebral movement

Transverse vertebral pressure against the tip of the transverse processes of C1, both towards the left and towards the right, was extremely sensitive to Grade I pressure.

Central postero-anterior vertebral pressure on C1 was equally tender, as were unilateral postero-anterior pressures on the left and on the right articular pillars at level C1, right more so than left.

Her X-rays were checked (cervical spine) and showed a narrowing of the left interlaminar space between the atlas and the axis (C1/C2)

Treatment

	//	
Five Grade I pressures were given at each of the joints identified by palpation	//	c/o Throbbing worse – for about sixty seconds and then to previous level Total head pain now reverted to cap pattern and less severe
The rest of the cervical articulations were palpated for tenderness and mobilized with Grade I pressures, increasing the number of pressures lower down. At C7, 15 × Grade I unilateral pressures were given on each side	//	
C4 central postero-anteriorly was very tender and was mobilized in the same way, postero-anteriorly, Grade I × 10 pressures	//	Headache as above
Manual longitudinal pull, Grade IV, 10 seconds	//	Throbbing less tinnitus gone neck pain now less feels dizzy
o/e Painful soft tissue thickening, suboccipital, was frictioned		

On the following day the patient said that after the treatment she had felt much better for the rest of the day and had not needed anything for the pain until that night.

Note: She had been due for her pain pills just before commencement of treatment, and the treatment obviated the need to take them.

The same treatment was given as that on the previous day. On the third visit she said that she was fine and had not had headache since the previous day but that her neck was a bit sore. On the fourth day she reported no recurrence of headache, no neck pain or dizziness or tinnitus.

Examination

Cervical physiological movement were all of full range and pain-free with overpressure except for right flexion at 7/8 range, left-sided neck pain and left upper cervical quadrant, left-sided neck pain.

The same treatment was repeated.

The next day she was to be discharged and I would not see her again as she lived far away. If she had been an outpatient attending my rooms I would, at this stage, have asked her to report back in a week's time and tailed off her treatment as explained in Chapter 11. But under the circumstances I decided to do a Grade V manipulation to the occipito-atlanto-axial joints in order to finally free them.

I repeated the usual treatment, increasing the grades to IIIs and IVs and then, after testing for vertebral artery patency, which was intact, did localized manipulations at O/C1/C2 levels.

Discussion

Although this patient was not able to be contacted for follow-up purposes, the case demonstrates many points described in this book.

A lesion was demonstrable on X-ray at C6/7. Radiological studies seldom show a lesion at C1/2, but frequently at C6/7, and so in post-whiplash headache cases the headache is commonly thought to arise at the lesion which is visible on X-ray. But although the low cervical lesion may be symptomatic and causing neck/scapular/arm pain, it is the upper cervical lesion which is referring pain to the head, even if it is not to be seen radiologically (*see* Chapter 4). I do not think that the lower lesion, in the absence of an upper cervical lesion, will give rise to headache but only to neck/scapular/arm pain. But when the lower as well as the upper lesions are symptomatic, both need to be treated before the headache will finally abate. It seems that the pain and paravertebral muscle spasm caused by the lower lesion will perpetuate the symptom of headache coming from the upper lesion until it too is cleared.

The escalating periodicity of the true cervical headache is clearly demonstrated in this case. The occasional headaches she describes in early adulthood indicate an early syndrome, which is common in many people who consider it to be normal. They might never have become any more than that if she had not walked into her cupboard door without ducking. After that incident, which was repeated, the condition became worse with a resulting escalation of symptoms. The periodicity, from **P = 1/5** (occasional) became **P = 3/5** (two or three times a week) and finally **P = 5/5** (continuous) with commensurate increase in intensity of pain and decrease in analgesic response.

TPP = 14/15

The final escalation of the syndrome resulted in her hospitalization, and, judging by the drug regimen, was diagnosed as status migrainosis. But neither the migraine-specific drugs nor the drugs prescribed to release nervous tension and so muscle spasm resulted in remission of pain. The cervical spine was X-rayed only because of the severe neck pain and, because there was a demonstrable lesion, was referred for physiotherapy.

The fact that accurate cervical mobilization immediately caused all the symptoms to abate demonstrates not only the correctness of the diagnosis resulting from radiological evidence, but the treatment chosen. But if, as is most commonly the case, there had been no radiologically demonstrable lesion, this patient might not have been referred for appropriate treatment.

The severity of the syndrome, or a long history of chronicity, do not mean that the condition will respond poorly, as is demonstrated here. The results obtained in this case, although dramatic, are not surprising to those of us who have learned to approach headaches in this way. In fact, because we so often have quick and easy results, we are too easily discouraged when they are slow to come and we have to work harder and longer for them.

It is usually not easy to get quick results with hospitalized patients, not because their condition is more severe, but because the conditions of total rest and drug management do not represent their usual lifestyle and so, when there is remission of pain it does not necessarily mean that the foregoing treatment of mobilization was what caused it. It is not easy to evaluate the efficacy of techniques. In this case it was possible to do so because the patient had been in hospital for a week on the drug regimen, with no abatement of headache, and so when the headache responded to the first treatment I knew that I should repeat whatever I had done on the day before. A headache which is intermittent, or erratic in its periodicity pattern, which is usually more difficult to treat than a continuous headache, is even more difficult to treat when the patient is hospitalized.

Case 8

A case of migraine for comparison with case histories of cervical headaches.

A 49-year-old woman told me that she had been a migraine sufferer for many years. The syndrome had started when she was a student. The pain, which is felt above the left eye and encroaching onto the base of the nose is of a deep dull character which builds up to a totally incapacitating intensity. The headache occurred episodically once every four to six months. She said that there could be remission periods of up to 18 months.

If she took a migraine-specific drug at the very onset and lay down in a dark room with an ice pack, she was able to abort it but it could return on the following day. Analgesics were quite ineffective.

Although the onset of attack was unpredictable, she thought that it was more likely to happen premenstrually or when she was under stress. It was worse when she was pregnant with her third child. Percolated coffee would usually result in a migraine attack, although there have been times when she could drink it with no ill effect.

The headache was preceded by some difficulty of focus in the form of a wavery visual disturbance. This was followed by neck spasm and at this stage pressure on the neck afforded a feeling of relief.

The severity of pain has been maximal since the onset of the syndrome and the periodicity has always varied from 1–18 months between attacks in a random and not a progressive manner.

She had consulted her general practitioner who referred her to an ophthalmologist. Extensive eye tests revealed no abnormality. She then saw a professor of neurology who carried out objective tests including a CT brain scan and no pathology was demonstrable. A diagnosis of migraine was arrived at and vasoconstrictor drugs were prescribed. She had been a motion-sick child but not an allergic one. There was no family history of migraine.

This condition did not respond to any other treatment applied to the cervical spine. The story is typical of the vascular migraine. See the examination chart for typical cervical headache in the Appendix and compare.

Appendix

Headache examination chart (This chart has been typeset here for clarity but would usually be filled in by hand)

1. Distribution

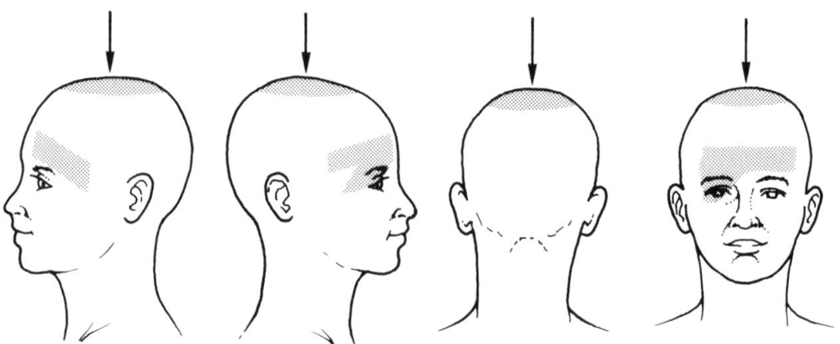

2. Description of pain

Inward pressure on vertex. Frontal pain steady, even.

3. Intensity (I) = 3/5

Moderate. Is 'able to function, when pain at its worst, without too much difficulty'.
*Intensity has worsened over past 2–3 years.

4. Periodicity (P) = 4/5

Every afternoon for the past 2 years . . . Before that, 2–3 days/week (P = 3/5).

No H/A until ± age 23, then occasional headache until 2 years ago, then daily.

Possible trauma when whiplash injury in adolescence
* Periodicity worsens.

5. Response to pain tablets (R) = 3/5

When I = 3/5, pain is abated by taking 2 compound analgesics. Previously, simple analgesics were effective but no longer.

$$\text{TPP} = \underset{(P)}{4/5} + \underset{(I)}{3/5} + \underset{(R)}{3/5} = 10/15$$

6. Aggravating or precipitating factors

Desk work. Headache comes on after midday (posture).
Deadlines or too much work (tension).
Car journeys (sustained position, glare, tension in traffic)

7. Associated symptoms

When I = 3/5, some blurring of vision. Nothing else.

8. Previous treatment

Muscle relaxant drugs – no benefit.
Compound analgesics/sedatives – temporary relief.
Physiotherapy – electrical (TENS, USR) massage – no benefit.
All neuro. objective tests done but negative.
Previous diagnosis – tension headache.

9. Points of interest

The only causative factor suggested is the M.V.A. (motor vehicle accident) in which she sustained a whiplash injury to her neck.

Conclusion

This worsening syndrome following trauma to the neck strongly suggests a cervicogenic articular headache. It has not yet reached its full development but, without appropriate treatment to the upper cervical spine (mobilization) it will continue to worsen to a TPP of

$$\frac{14\text{–}15}{15}$$

There is nothing here to suggest vascular migraine.

Tentative diagnosis

Post traumatic cervical headache – diagnosis will be confirmed if mobilization of cervical spine reduces the TPP from 10/15 to 3/15.

Index